The Art and Science of Personalising Care with Older People with Diabetes

Trisha Dunning
Editor

The Art and Science of Personalising Care with Older People with Diabetes

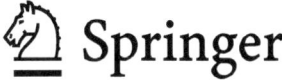 Springer

Editor
Trisha Dunning
Barwon Health
Deakin University Barwon Health
Geelong
Victoria
Australia

ISBN 978-3-030-08972-6   ISBN 978-3-319-74360-8   (eBook)
https://doi.org/10.1007/978-3-319-74360-8

Printed on acid-free paper

This Springer imprint is published by the registered company Springer International Publishing AG part of Springer Nature
The registered company address is: Gewerbestrasse 11, 6330 Cham, Switzerland

Foreword

I have known Professor Trisha Dunning for more than 20 years but met face to face with her for the first time in Vancouver at an International Diabetes Federation (IDF) meeting. We were sharing the platform for a symposium on the very substance of this book, *diabetes in older people*! It was then that I appreciated how compassionate an individual she is about wishing to improve the lot of this often vulnerable and neglected population of people with diabetes. She introduced the idea that we, as a caring group of professionals, must listen more to what our patients are saying, take a greater interest in each of their life histories, and try to 'personalise' care at every opportunity. Her use of case histories was memorable. Her talk not surprisingly was received best out of all three speakers! I realised we shared similar concerns about the inadequacies and inequity of diabetes care of older people and since then we have been actively collaborating—which has been a privilege and honour for me!

There are few people in the world of diabetes care who have won the admiration and respect afforded to Trisha. She has been an inspirational leader for nearly two decades, always pushing the agenda for change and improvement in care in those highly important and challenging areas that still receive less attention than they warrant such as care home diabetes, end of life diabetes care, and pharmacovigilance.

Trisha is already an accomplished academic, researcher, and writer of textbooks, and so you might think that the development of this new book might have seemed straightforward for her. This thought was never in her mind, however, because she knew it had to be different from other books available in this area, as well as thought provoking, being able to motivate health professionals and others to go out there and make a difference to the lives of their patients, and of real clinical utility—this book accomplishes all of these aims.

The book comprises ten chapters, half of which are written by Trisha and the other five written by accomplished writers and scientists, most of whom are active locally and therefore on the same wavelength for creating this exciting new book. The term 'personalised care' is often taken for granted and may be considered 'stereotyped'! However, this book unlocks the real meaning of this term and how it should be applied to modern diabetes care of older people in our society. The book explains what the key aims of care should be, how shared decision-making and holistic care are fundamental to achieve meaningful outcomes, and how clinical guidelines can assist in personalising care but at the same time stressing how this concept must be an essential part of future guideline developments. With chapters on technology, life transitions, nutritional therapy, the challenges of dementia, and future research directions, the book is complete and still remarkably concise. As the title of the book implies, both artistic merit and scientific rigour underpin the principal drive that this book has required.

You should read this book if you want to enhance your own clinical experience in managing the aged individual with diabetes as the process of 'personalisation' will reveal how complex an illness it can be and how routine care has its major shortcomings. It will also stimulate your interest to recognise that many older people do indeed have unique life experiences that will affect their attitudes and responses to your treatment plans. By reading the book, you will be able to motivate others, perhaps members of your interdisciplinary team, to take on board the principles embodied in this short treatise that define and justify the importance of personalised care.

Birmingham, UK   Alan Sinclair, M.Sc., M.D., F.R.C.P.

Preface

The wisdom and experience of older people is a resource of inestimable worth. Recognising and treasuring the contributions of older people is essential to the long term flourishing of any society.

Daisaku Ikeda (2007)

A colleague asked: *Where did this book come from?*, which caused me to reflect on where and how did originate—besides the fact I am an older person with a vested interest in advocating for the care of older people with diabetes.

My respect for older people and love of stories began in my early childhood. We lived on an isolated bush property when I was very young. There was no electricity, street lights, telephones, or close neighbours. Dad grew most of our fruit and vegetables and we made a long trek into town for groceries and other necessities once a month. When I turned five I went to live with my Grandma and Pop so I could go to school. Grandma and Pop moved to town from their farm a few years before. Pop developed dementia shortly after they moved and often wandered down the street and stood beneath the street lights quietly watching the 'fairies' (insects) and rainbows around the light. It was my job to bring him home.

Grandma was a stoical, hardworking, no nonsense woman who had some great sayings that influenced who I am: for example *A whistling woman is good to neither God nor man.* I never had the courage to ask her what a whistling woman *was* good for! She was adamant that ladies *do not wear dangling earrings—other kinds of women, like gypsies, do that.* I cannot whistle, and I have never worn dangling earrings. I am not sure what that makes me good for, or whether I am a lady!

One day Grandma was ill and unable to care for me for a few weeks. I went to live with her sister, my Great Aunt Lizzie and my Great Grandma (Nana) in Aunt Lizzie's wonderful house and cottage garden. Aunt Lizzie taught me to cook and enhanced my love of gardening. Both women inadvertently introduced me to the fact that old people die.

Nana was bitten by a snake while she was picking thistles for her canaries. Aunt Lizzie found her several hours later 'dozing in the sun'. Nana often dosed in the sun so I did not realise she died, until much later—she was dozing and was taken away. Aunt Lizzie died in hospital 2 years later. My father would not let me visit her because it would upset me to *'see her like that'*. I still do not know *'what like that'* actually meant, and I still carry unresolved grief at not being able to say goodbye to her. These old ladies and my Mum shared their accumulated wisdom and taught me compassion and respect.

When I started nursing I encountered vulnerable older people reliant on care to survive. I nursed older people with dementia who were often violent or verbally abusive—a stark contrast to the self-caring, independent women in my family and my docile Pop with dementia. There were no aged care homes or supported accommodation in the town, so dependent older people lived in the hospital if their families were not able to care for them.

Diabetes was rare in those days, or perhaps unrecognised: some people with cardiovascular disease and stroke probably also had diabetes. We had few medicines to treat diabetes apart from Metformin, Glibenclamide, and animal insulins that were administered using large glass syringes and long needles that had to be sharpened and sterilised after each use. There were no blood glucose meters. Initially we tested urine for glucose using Fehling's solution and eventually Clinitest tablets. There was no test for ketones, except the smell of new mown hay. Diabetes self-care was unheard of.

I learned a lot about diabetes and witnessed many advances in diabetes care over the years that improved outcomes, quality of life, and life expectancy for people with diabetes. These changes improved diabetes care and led to diabetes self-management programmes. They also increased self-care and treatment burdens that added to the disease and medicine burden for older people with functional and cognitive changes that lower their resilience to stressors.

Most of my research over the past 10 years concerned care of older people with diabetes and was undertaken *with* advisory groups of older people with diabetes and their families, whose wisdom and life and diabetes experience, which they so generously share, enhance my research and the applicability of the findings to diabetes clinical practice.

These factors are the impetus for and origin of my belief in person-centred care: the core concept underpinning the book. The idea for the book emerged following a conversation with Nathalie Lhorset-Poulain from Springer, after a workshop I delivered with colleagues at the 2015 International Diabetes Federation Congress in Vancouver. I am very grateful to her for her interest and support.

The Preface is not the ramblings of a garrulous old woman. There are important messages in the snippets of my story shared in this Preface. The story is an important reminder that all older people were once young. They are highly individual. They all have stories. They all have explanatory models for many things, including diabetes. We can only truly understand the *person* and plan care *with* them if we look beyond their age and their diabetes and see the person. We can only see the person if we are prepared to hear their stories.

Reading literature forces readers to *fill in gaps and search for meanings among a spectrum of possible meanings* (Bruner 1986). One reason Drs. Cookson and Holmes insisted we read literary stories as well as nursing/medical texts was to enhance our capacity to relate to the people we cared for and their social situation.

References

Bruner J (1986) Actual minds. Possible worlds. Harvard University, Cambridge, MA, p 25

Daisaku Ikeda (2007) Realising the potential of an ageing society. The Japan Times March 8

Geelong, Australia   Trisha Dunning

Acknowledgements

Many people inspired and contributed to this book. I acknowledge two general practitioners, Dr. Charles Cookson and Dr. Charles Holmes, who were mentors and tutors over the 4 years of my nursing training. They taught at teachable moments and not strictly according to the order of curriculum. They took us on home visits and to post-mortems; they insisted we read novels as well as nursing and medical texts. Their supportive teaching style that incorporated art and science was ahead of its time and much of what I learned is reflected in the book.

More recently, colleagues from Barwon Health and Deakin University, Dr. Mark Kennedy who often acts as a sounding board for my ideas, and international colleagues, especially Professor Alan Sinclair, colleague and friend for over 10 years, influenced this book—although they might not know it!

I am grateful to my co-authors, Bodil, Mark, Sital, David, and Natalie, for agreeing to contribute to the book and for writing such great chapters. Their expertise adds depth and value to the book.

Most of all, I acknowledge the many people with diabetes who taught me so much about living with diabetes by sharing their experiences, stories, and explanatory models over the years. I love working with advisory groups of people with diabetes on my research projects; their advice is invaluable.

I am grateful to the Publisher, Springer, especially Nathalie Lhorset-Poulain, who initiated the book, and Abha Krishnan, who monitored the book production.

I owe a very big thank you to Professor Alan Sinclair for writing the foreword to this book and for his friendship and advice.

I acknowledge Indigenous Cultures whose knowledge was largely transmitted orally as stories/songlines. Indigenous people were able to commit a vast amount of information about their culture, practices, and the land to memory. Survival depended on knowing where food and water could be obtained as well as custodianship of the land. Australian Indigenous songlines, stored in memory and passed from generation-to-generation, extend across the country. The method of remembering, recently daubed 'the memory code', is being adopted by teachers in some Australian schools. I particularly acknowledge the Wauthaurang people, on whose land most of this book was written.

My very special thanks go to my husband, John, for his unfailing support—he is the wind beneath my wings. I received a great deal of 'help' from our two beautiful West Highland White Terriers, Flora Weadora and MacBeth MacDunning. I could not have written the book without Flora's help with word processing, her cuddles, and her attentive listening (Like a Dog) as I read the book out loud. MacBeth, a frail old man who slept a lot and kept my feet warm during the writing process, died 2 weeks before the book was submitted to the publisher. He taught me a lot about cherishing and caring for older people.

Contents

Overview of Older People, Ageing and Diabetes, the Disease

Trisha Dunning

[A volunteer in an aged care home for veterans] spent two hours listening to one of the ladies on the lawn talk about working for Ziegfeld. Afterward the woman apologized profoundly for 'boring you with my stories.' Vivian could have listened for two more hours and not realized time going by. These people were not just old veterans. They were living history books dismissed by almost everyone stupid enough to think they were not worth reading.

(Callahan 2015)

Key Points

- Older people are individuals: they are not defined by their age or their diabetes.
- Ageing is unique to every individual. Chronological age is not a good indicator of health status or care needs.
- Health status in older age is influenced by genetics and lifestyle behaviours in younger age.
- Increasing age is a risk factor for diabetes. Most older people have type 2 diabetes but people with type 1 diabetes survive to older age and type 1 can be first diagnosed in older age.
- It is essential to personalise care *with* the individual and to use a proactive, risk identification and minimise approach.

T. Dunning, A.M., M.Ed., Ph.D., R.N., C.D.E.
Centre for Quality and Patient Safety Research, Barwon Health Partnership,
Deakin University, Geelong, VIC, Australia
e-mail: trisha.dunning@barwonhealth.org.au;
trisha.dunning@deakin.edu.au

© Springer International Publishing AG, part of Springer Nature 2018
T. Dunning (ed.), *The Art and Science of Personalising Care with Older People with Diabetes*, https://doi.org/10.1007/978-3-319-74360-8_1

1.1   Introduction

This chapter outlines older age and diabetes to set the context for the other chapters in the book. Detailed information about diabetes pathophysiology and management can be found in the guidelines, position statements and reference texts listed in the recommended reading at the end of the chapter.

The global population is ageing and the post-World War 2 generation, the 'Baby Boomers', have very different expectations, preferences and values about their older age than previous generations. The Australian Centre for Social Innovation (tacsi) (2016) identified the following 'big themes' from interviews with baby boomers. They:

- Believe they need to keep working to pay the bills.
- Want to stay in their own homes and grow old where they are known and where their connections are.
- Have very different expectations of health services, including aged care services.
- Feel it is important to 'keep young in the mind'.
- Do not want 'currently available' aged care services, especially ending up in an aged care home, but realise they may need help when they can no longer self-care.

These are not particularly new findings. Lansky identified similar themes/concerns in 1998 in the USA. These were to:

- Be treated with respect.
- Understand what they are told.
- Have access to the health services and providers they need.
- Stay healthy as long as possible, which included having access to education, preventative services and early diagnosis of disease.
- Recover from illnesses and regain normal functioning.
- Live with their illness if they have a chronic disease.
- Be able to cope with changing needs and death and disability in their family by treating pain and suffering.

These findings suggest older people have a basically realistic but positive attitude to their ageing, which differs from the National Ageing Research Institute (NARI) report (2017). The NARI report suggested many countries use a 'doom and gloom', pervasively negative ageing narratives and suggested the language should be changed to positive, inclusive language because if people are consistently given negative messages about older age they begin to believe they have no value. NARI indicate positive messages are particularly important to the 'new middle age' (50–75 years) who have increasing life expectancy, the rapidly changing global social and economic climates.

Many countries have adopted various 'ageing' strategies/frameworks to support people as they grow older and help them 'age in place' in their own homes or in the community for as long as possible. These frameworks include:

- Active ageing
- Healthy ageing
- Successful ageing
- Reablement/restorative care

Most ageing frameworks and strategies are based on the need to support physical and cognitive function as well as economic imperatives, social needs, and the person's capacity to engage with life and other people. New technology such as the five good friends app, Facebook and Skype help older people remain connected (see Chap. 9).

It is difficult to define 'successful ageing'. One size does not fit every older person. Therefore, it is important to ask the individual what 'successful ageing' means to them; or better still, not use the term, given the alternative, 'failed ageing', is very negative!

Older people develop creative ways to remain independent and preserve their dignity; for example, friends living independently on the same site with some shared facilities such as gardens. Despite these positive initiatives, the demand for formal home care, aged care home services is increasing in most countries due to the ageing population and societal changes such as family structure and lifestyle that affect family caregiving capacity (Weng and Landes 2017). Thus, care is often provided by lay 'health aids'.

In addition, many countries are culturally and linguistically diverse, which can lead to communication, engagement and connection issues. Different individuals and cultures have different explanatory models for health, care, ageing and diabetes. These diverse similarities and differences lead to the question: who are older people?

1.2 Older People

'Older' age is commonly defined as older than age 65 (World Health Organisation (WHO) 2002, 2017). Some older people, including older health professionals, indicate 'the older one gets, the older old is', and state 'you are only as old as you feel', as the following anecdote shows:

> *I am going to my writing group, now.*
> *OK. Who will be there?*
> *Mostly older people—retired teachers.*
> *So, one more older person will join them—you!!*

Chronological age is not a good indicator of personhood, health status or function and it is not a useful basis on which to plan care. Older people are highly individual; therefore it is essential to consider each person's physical, mental and spiritual, functional status and life expectancy when planning care (Dunning et al. 2013; IDF 2013; Sinclair et al. 2014). Spirituality is an important life dimension and is concerned with finding meaning and purpose in life and the events people encounter throughout their lives (see Chap. 7). Key dimensions of spirituality include relationships with self and others. It may or may not include religion.

Each older person is an individual and has unique life experiences, inherited characteristics and social circumstances. Older people have sexual health needs, which are often not addressed. Some develop sexually transmitted disease, some are homeless, some are abused, and some are alcoholics. Some travel a lot. Most have a significant body of accumulated wisdom and learned patterns associated with their life, their diabetes and self-care that help them cope with their diabetes, life and other health problems in older age.

However, changed circumstances and uncertainty can cause stress and increase cognitive load, which affect self-care, pattern recognition, problem-solving and self-confidence, especially during illnesses. Importantly, older individual's unique values, preferences, life goals and their opinions must be identified as part of comprehensive assessments and respected; otherwise it is impossible to develop personalised care plans.

It is essential to tailor care to suit the individual (personalised care). In order to personalise care, professionals must understand ageing, diabetes and their cumulative effects on physical and cognitive function, and have impeccable communication skills and cultivate the art of eliciting older people's stories to collaboratively develop care plans *with* the older individual, and sometimes their family carers (see Chaps. 2 and 3). Personalised care must encompass general health and social care as well as diabetes care and be regularly reviewed. People's stories need to be viewed in the context of their whole life.

1.3   Ageism and Stereotyping

Ageist attitudes and stereotypical, discriminatory language is common in the general population, the media and in health care. Ageism refers to discrimination because of older age. The focus is often on the negative aspects of ageing, less often on the positive aspects such as wisdom and patience. Stereotyping occurs when characteristics associated with age are applied to all older people (Butler 1969, 1980). NARI (2017) highlighted the need to use positive rather than negative 'old age' language.

Negative ageism is disrespectful to the individual and their family and has negative effects on older people's self-esteem and health outcomes (Richeson and Shelton 2006). Significantly, it is not consistent with personalised care or shared decision-making. Research shows 'elderspeak' leads to cognitively impaired older people adopting resistive behaviours during care provision. Elderspeak refers to babytake and using words such as 'darl', 'lovey' and other depersonalising and demeaning language. When elderspeak was modified to more respectful language, resistive behaviour was significantly reduced (REF).

1.4   What Is 'Old Age?'

Old age is not a status we choose to become; it is a status that we inherit simply by the virtue of living, not dying. (Holstein 2006)

As indicated, 'old age' generally refers to people older than age 65 (WHO 2002, 2017). Chronological age refers to the linear passage of time from birth onwards and is understood as *chronos* time. *Chronos* time is quantitative and refers to duration of time (Mc Fadden and Thibault 2001). It is useful to maintain schedules, understand disease progression and plan for future care. However, chronological age does not necessarily reflect an individual's biological age, their functional capacity or their perceived age, and is not the best indicator of their care needs or their potential lifespan.

Another time dimension, *kairos* time, refers to opportunity or a suitable time to take action (Mc Fadden and Thibault 2001). That is, 'in the moment time' and 'decision time' (*seize the day*). *Kairos* time is qualitative and is experienced in the moment when people are engaged in immediate experiences, often when decisive action is needed. *Kairos* timed is meaningful for individuals and their connections (Mc Fadden and Thibault 2001). There are many *kairos* moments in an individual's life journey besides those associated with diabetes.

An individual's life journey moves through both dimensions of time. Older people are often focused on maintaining meaning and purpose in their life, being connected and maintaining hope. They are important to quality of life and survival, in combination with 'a healthy lifestyle'.

Many older people, including those with diabetes, are self-caring and live in the community. Some require various degrees of support to undertake Activities of Daily Living (ADL) and/or Instrumental Activities of Daily Living (IADL). A great deal of support is provided by family members. Between 25 and 30% of older people living in care homes have diabetes (Sinclair et al. 2001; Anderson 2014) and a further 25% are undiagnosed but at risk of diabetes (Dunning et al. 2013; Anderson 2014) and may not receive adequate treatment, which could affect well-being, comfort and quality of life.

The combination of diabetes, comorbidities and dementia lead to the individual needing increasingly complex care. Carers need to be able to recognise and manage changes such as hypo- and hyperglycaemia and their effects on well-being, cognition and self-care capacity.

1.5 Factors That Influence Longevity

Life expectancy has increased due to environmental improvements in food and water, control of communicable disease, and technological advances in medical care that enable a range of life-limiting illnesses, including cardiovascular disease and cancer, to be effectively managed for long periods of time. Conversely, technology also contributed to the increase in obesity-related diseases that reduce life expectancy, e.g. by reducing the amount of physical activity needed to catch and prepare food.

Box 1.1 outlines the recommendations for healthy living proposed by ancient healers and philosophers. These recommendations still apply today. Interestingly, Aretaeus, who practised medicine in 120 AD, wrote,

The condition [diabetes] *is fortunately rare but short will be the life of the man in whom the disease is fully developed.* (King et al. 1999)

Box 1.1: Recommendations About Old Age in Ancient Cultures

Modern ageing research largely supports the following recommendations of ancient philosopher and healers such as Cicero, Plato, Solon, and Hippocrates (Dunning 2017). Their recommendations still make common and 'clinical' sense today.

- Growing older is normal and inevitable: not a disease.
- Individuals age at different rates and the speed at which an individual and their individual tissues and organs age depends on humours. These 'humours', hot, cold, dry and wet, influence body function. If the humours became unbalanced, ill health occurs. Modern genomics, epigenetics and other 'nomics' may be a modern way to explain ancient 'balance theories'.
- Older people were encouraged to plan for their older age while they were 'young', including planning for their end of life. Age 50 was old, until relatively recently and is still old in some underprivileged societies. 'Old age' as now defines as older than 65 years (WHO 2002). Many older people do not regard themselves as old (Richeson and Shelton 2006).
- A healthy diet and regular exercise contribute to a healthy old age.
- Learning something new every day throughout life is essential to brain health.
- People were expected to contribute to society. Today many older people contribute to society and the economy through paid and volunteer work, including caring for older family members.
- Society has a collective and individual responsibility to care for its older people.

Diabetes is extremely common today, despite primary prevention strategies and knowledge about the associated devastating complications. Consequently, the second statement is as true today as it was in 120 AD. Most people with diabetes develop complications that reduce life expectancy. Type 2 diabetes is a progressive, incurable disease and complications are present in up to 50% of people with type 2 diabetes, even at the time of diagnosis (King et al. 1999).

Ageing is a gradual process. Age is the biggest risk factor for some of the most debilitating diseases known and feared today such as neurodegenerative diseases, Alzheimer's disease, cardiovascular disease, and inflammatory and metabolic diseases such as diabetes and cancer. Most of these comorbidities are associated with diabetes. Older people often have 3–5 coexisting comorbidities that need to be co-managed. Some studies focus on understanding and preventing/curing ageing as a way to reverse the pathogenesis of several diseases: for example, identifying the predictors of physiological age and developing new medicines to that target the physiological processes associated with ageing.

Ageing and longevity are moderated by genetic and non-genetic factors and many biological and biochemical mechanisms. Genetic factors account for 25% of the variation in longevity (Passarino et al. 2016). Studies into the genetic and molecular basis of ageing identified several genes associated with maintaining cells and basic cell metabolism that affect individual variation in the ageing phenotype.

Some genes are protective and confer greater functional reserves. Genes involved in lipoprotein metabolism, especially APOE, cardiovascular homeostasis, immunity and inflammation play a role in ageing, age-related disorders and longevity (Schachtner et al. 1994). Ageing is also associated with mitochondrial dysfunction and changes in metabolic function (Lopez-Otin et al. 2013; Petersen et al. 2004).

Alzheimer's disease is one of the most feared diseases associated with old age. People with T2DM are at risk of cognitive impairment, structural changes in the brain and brain atrophy (Rizzo et al. 2010; Launer et al. 2011).The pathogenesis of Alzheimer's disease commences decades before the onset of symptoms present. People who carry the APOE E4 allele are at increased risk of Alzheimer's disease while the E2 allele has a protective effect (Sun et al. 2012). Recently, HealthWatch, a nutritional genomics company that studies gene-diet disease interactions, launched HealthWatch 360 (www.gbhealthwatch.com/healthwatch360-app/) to provide nutrition advice to help people manage their Alzheimer's risk.

HealthWatch 360 also offers people the opportunity of finding out their genetic risk of Alzheimer's based on their APOE genotype. APOE e4 has high sensitivity and high positive predictive value for the diagnosis of Alzheimer's disease but a low negative predictive value and specificity. APOE genotyping may help diagnose the condition, especially when people have atypical signs or early age onset of dementia (Sun et al. 2012). Chapter 8 discusses caring for older people with cognitive impairment and dementia in more detail.

Imagine how Alice, a 50-year-old Harvard linguistics professor recently diagnosed with early onset Alzheimer's disease, felt when she said:

> *I can see the words hanging in front of me and I can't reach them, and I don't know who I am, and I don't know what I'm going to lose next.* (Genova 2009)

Chronic inflammation has a negative impact on tissues and organs and is a consequence of glucose variability as well as chronic hyperglycaemia (Kovalchev and Cobelli 2016). Glucose variability refers to excursions/fluctuations between high and low blood glucose. Fluctuations can be measure by time and by amplitude. The mean amplitude of the glucose excursions (MAGE) is an important determinant of overall metabolic status and risk of complications.

MAGE is significantly associated Mini Mental State Examination (MMSE) scores and composite scores of cognition, independently of age, gender, Body Mass

Index (BMI), waist-hip ratio, medicines and physical activity, which highlights the need to consider MAGE as well as HbA1c when deciding management strategies. Continuous glucose monitoring enables glucose variations to be measured in real time and is becoming used more frequently in diabetes self-care and in acute care settings such as intensive care units.

Low grade inflammation, after age, is the most important determinant of capability, cognition and survival (Ari et al. 2015). Recent research suggests preventing hyperglycaemia is important in older people. It is not a benign condition. The challenge is to balance the adverse consequences of hyperglycaemia with the devastating effects of hypoglycaemia, which includes falls and mortality risk.

Studies show genes associated with the pathways involved in nutrient signalling and regulating transcription factors such as IGF-1/insulin axis and TOR modulate longevity (Junnila et al. 2013). Animal studies show that molecules that modulate these pathways prevent a range of age-related diseases such as cancer, cardiovascular disease, osteoporosis and T2DM. Research is underway to determine whether medicines can modulate these pathways and slow human ageing, in particular, activating a key sirtuin, SIRTI (Hubbard and Sinclair 2014). Sirtuin is one of the silent information regulator genes that promote longevity in many species and mediate the beneficial effects of restricting calories.

More recently, epigenetic studies show that epigenetic changes modulated by genetic inheritance and lifestyle are sensitive to ageing and could be a biomarker of ageing or influence the ageing and/or rate and quality of the ageing process. Horvath et al. formulated a mathematical model to predict an individual's chronological age from the methylation levels of several body cells and tissues based on their work on the Epigenome-wide Association Studies.

The so-called epigenetic clock or Horvath's clock may be an accurate biomarker of age, superior to estimates based on telomere length and can predict all-cause mortality after adjusting for traditional risk factors (Horvath 2013). Interestingly, studies in supercentenarians show the brain and muscle are the youngest body tissues in these individuals (Wagner 2017). It is not clear how widely the epigenetic clock is applied to prognostication outside research and its relevance to clinical care or palliative and end of life care planning is unclear.

Genes and small molecules involved in maintaining DNA repair (Debrabant et al. 2014), conserving telomeres (Sorensen et al. 2012), the heat shock response, and managing free radical levels (Raule et al. 2016) influence longevity. Function is reduced if these processes are not maintained and cellular ageing is accelerated through DNA methylation. Three main pathways control lifespan in mammals: insulin/IGF-1, TSCn/TOR and sirtuins (Hubbard and Sinclair 2014). The latter are central to the body's response to diet and exercise. These three pathways possibly control the response to adversity and cellular stress that contributes to DNA damage and hypoxia. Many of the biomarkers that drive ageing and the functional and pathological changes that result can be measured as shown in Box 1.2.

Box 1.2: Some Functional and Physiological Measures of Age-Related Changes
- Haematopoiesis/anaemia
- Oxidative changes that reflect inflammation
- Blood lipid and blood glucose
- Liver and renal function
- Cell and immune senescence
- DEXA
- Bone Mineral density
- Barthel Index (ADL)
- Lowton Index (IADL)
- Morbidity count
- Cognitive function MMSE
- Life expectancy—Mortality—survival score
- Estimates of frailty such as Grip strength, gait speed and walking distance

Humane endogenous retroviruses, HERVs or fossil viruses, are present in approximately 8% of the human genome. HERVs originated from ancestral infections in the germ line during millions of years of evolution and have been inherited by successive generations (Nelson et al. 2003; Zanh et al. 2015). HERVs might confer biological benefits. There are implicated in some cancers, autoimmune diseases such as rheumatoid arthritis, Systemic Lupus Erythematosus and Type 1 diabetes but the association with Type 1 diabetes in not confirmed (Nelson et al.2003).

1.6 Diabetes and Ageing

The two main types of diabetes: type 1 an autoimmune disease and type 2 a progressive disease associated with declining beta cell function both occur in older people, although type 2 is the most common. Figure 1.1 outlines basic glucose homeostasis.

Older age is a risk factor for diabetes due to age-related pathophysiological changes that affect glucose homeostasis, genetic predisposition, immune function and environmental risk factors (Meneilly 2011; IDF 2013; Munshi et al. 2016). Research demonstrates that keeping blood glucose as close to normal as possible reduces macro- and microvascular complications associated with hyperglycaemia (Diabetes Control and Complications Trial (DCCT) 1993; Turner et al. 1997; United Kingdom Prospective Study (UKPDS) 1998) and has a lasting or legacy effect up to 30 years later (Nathan et al. (DCCT/EDIC) 2014).

Ageing results in loss of beta cell mass and reduced capacity to regenerate the pancreatic beta cells, which leads to reduced insulin secretion, impaired glucose tolerance and hyperglycaemia. These are hallmarks of T2DM. Genetic predisposition

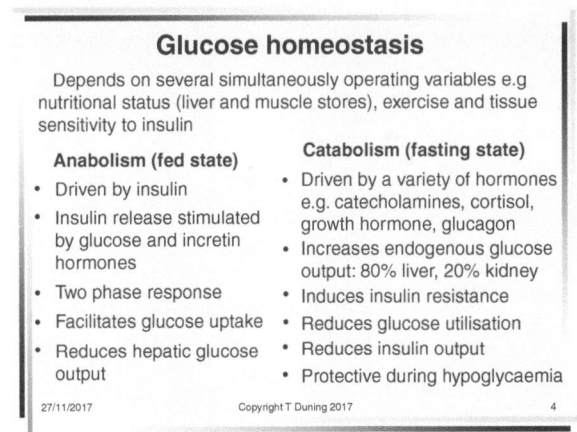

Fig. 1.1 Overview of glucose homeostasis

and lifestyle factors such as obesity and inactivity contribute to insulin resistance and loss of lean body mass (Hambling et al. 2016). Loss of lean body mass (sarcopenia) increases the risk of and frailty and its adverse consequences such as falls (Do-Yeon et al. 2016). Significantly, sarcopenia begins in middle age (REF).

Obesity and ageing contribute to the development of proinflammatory cytokines such as C-reactive protein, Inteleukin-6 and TFN alpha, which affect insulin signalling and increase insulin resistance and are associated with T2DM (Do-Yeon et al. 2016). Insulin signalling can be improved with regular activity, which also helps maintain blood glucose and lipids within an acceptable range and reduces inflammatory processes that lead to tissue damage. Hyperglycaemia is associated with micro- and macrovascular and neuropathic changes that affect the individual's ability to remain active and undertake Activities of Daily Living (ADL), Instrumental Activities of Daily Living (IADL) and diabetes self-care.

The role of the gut in glucose homeostasis through the incretin hormones is now well established and incretin hormone medications are available (Chap. 5). Recent research suggests there is an association between the gut microbiome and diabetes: in fact, altered gut microbiome could predict T2DM. The connection between the gut microbiota, glucose homeostasis could occur by altering fatty acid metabolism in the liver and adipose tissues, which contributes to low grade inflammation, obesity and insulin resistance in animal studies (Karlsson et al. 2013). Karlsson et al. (2013) showed particular bacterial species in the gut microbiome can differentiate between normal and abnormal glucose tolerance with similar predictive accuracy as traditional risk models, but the bacterial species most predictive of T2DM differs among ethnic groups.

In addition, new research suggests neurocircuits in a brain-centred glucoregulatory system play a role in glucose homeostasis by working with the beta cells in the pancreas in insulin-dependent ways and independently of insulin (Scarletti and Schwartz 2015). Some insulin-independent processes are activated by signals from the gut. Scarletti and Schwartz (2015) proposed a 'gut-brain-liver' axis for glucose homeostasis.

1.7   Overview of Diabetes

Diabetes is a chronic, progressive, incurable disease. Diabetes is now the most common disease in modern society and the prevalence is increasing (Ogurtsova et al. 2017). In 2015 an estimated 415 million people aged 20–79 years had diabetes; 5 million deaths were attributable to diabetes and the total global expenditure on diabetes was an estimated 673 billion USD. It is possible to live a long life with diabetes and this achievement is celebrated in countries such as the USA and Australia. Australia awards the Kellion Medal to people who survive 50 years with diabetes and the Victory Medal to people with type 1 diabetes who survive 80 years.

Most diabetes occurs in low- and middle-income countries. The prevalence in older people is over 20% in many countries with a further 20% at risk and undiagnosed. Likewise, between 20 and 30% of older people in care homes have diabetes (Sinclair et al. 2001; Anderson 2014).

Modern management means people with type 1 diabetes often live to older age. However, T1DM can be first diagnosed in older age. The basic management of both T1DM and T2DM is similar, diet, exercise and often medicines, with some important differences. People with T1DM depend on insulin to survive. Inadequate documentation of the type of diabetes in health records can lead to inappropriate withholding insulin and preventable ketoacidosis in older people withT1DM.

People with diabetes often have three to five diabetes complications and other comorbidities such as arthritis that affect their quality of life, functional status, and life expectancy (Meneilly 2011; IDF 2014; Munshi et al. 2016). Sexual health and well-being are important, but relatively neglected aspects, of care of older people and are part of psychological health. People with diabetes sexual heath can be affected by micro- and macrovascular disease, neuropathy, low mental health and some medicines.

Medicines are usually required to manage diabetes and its complications and other comorbidities; thus polypharmacy is common: thoughtful prescribing and pharmacovigilance are imperative (Dunning and Sinclair 2014), see Chap. 6. Significant complications result from micro- and macrovascular disease and sensory changes.

1.8   Microvascular Disease

Common microvascular diseases include retinopathy, renal disease and nephropathy. They affect self-care, driving, and independence and contribute to falls risk. Kirkman et al. (2012) suggested microvascular disease is a predictor of falls in people older than 80 years with T1DM. Other age-related eye diseases such as macular degeneration, cataract and glaucoma also affect independence and falls risk and driving safety and need to be assessed regularly.

Declining renal function has a significant effect on medicine choices, and life expectancy can lead to end stage renal disease and dialysis treatment. Recently,

Peters et al. (2017) described that Promarker D, a type of protein 'fingerprint', can predict kidney disease. Davis et al. claimed Promarker D was more accurate than commonly used tests of renal function such as eGFR and albumin excretion rate (ACR). Promarker D is not yet in common use in clinical practice.

Vision impairment affects the type of written and online information likely to be useful to older people including the content design features and language and literacy level. Hearing impairment can compromise communication and safety. Ensuring the person has their glasses and hearing aids during consultations and education sessions is essential to achieve an effective therapeutic relationship and cogenerate a care plan.

Foot disease is a consequence of microvascular and neuropathic disease as well as inadequate foot self-care. Serious infection can be present with few symptoms in people with neuropathy (Foster 2017). HPs have an important role providing foot education, inspecting the person's feet and protecting their feet from friction and pressure during emergency and hospital admissions. HPs also play an important role managing dialysis, screening for dental caries and depression in people with renal disease (National Institute of clinical Excellence (NICE) 2015).

1.9 Macrovascular Disease

Cardiovascular disease is the leading cause of death in people with diabetes. A recent US study examined BMI, diet, total cholesterol and blood pressure in 8961 children aged between 2 and 11 years. No child had ideal values for all four criteria. The findings support the contention that behaviours while young influences health in older age.

Cardiovascular health is also important to maintain nutrition and oxygen to the brain and maintain brain function. It is important to keep blood glucose close to the normal range and to avoid glucose variability from diagnosis. Near normal blood glucose can be risky for older people because it predisposes them to hypoglycaemia (McCoy et al. 2016). Managing hypertension, blood lipids and renal disease continues to be important in older people.

Generally, the recommended target blood pressure (BP) is <140/90 mmHg but may be 130/80 mmHg if it can be achieved without causing postural hypotension, which is associated with falls risk. Systolic BP < 130 and diastolic <75 mmHg may increase the mortality risk (ref). Antihypertensive and lipid lowering medicines and ACE inhibitors are often needed (British National Formulary https://www.scribd.com/document/.../British-National-Formulary-BNF-70-pdf; Australian Medicines Handbook 2017).

1.10 Type 2 Diabetes and the Brain

Age, diabetes, hypertension, chronic cardiovascular disease and the number of medicines people are using are all associated with brain atrophy to varying degrees. The effect of age on the brain is significant. The cumulative burden of cardiovascular risk factors from childhood are associated with reduced midlife cognitive performance (Yaffe et al. 2014) that may continue to decline in later life.

Rates of cortical activity are almost double in people aged 65–75 compared to those younger than 65. Animal and some human studies show chronic hyperglycaemia and glucose variability are possible links between T2DM and central nervous system (CNS) dysfunction (McCall 1992) mediated by the metabolic derangements caused by hyperglycaemia such as reduced regional cerebral blood flow, effects on the neurotransmitters adrenalin, dopamine and serotonin, and transporting glucose and choline (a precursor of acetylcholine) across the blood brain barrier. The latter is particularly relevant to memory. There is a strong link between memory disorders and acetylcholine.

Chronic hyperglycaemia triggers the development of advanced glycated end products (AGE), which damage vascular and other tissues and play a significant role in the development of diabetes-related complications. AGEs accumulate in the hippocampus during ageing and have been associated with the senile plaques and neurofibrillary tangles characteristic of Alzheimer's disease. Hyperglycaemia is also associated with increased aldose reductase activity, which results in accumulation of sorbitol, depletes myoinositol and alters Na-K ATPase activity, which disrupts transport of micronutrients into the central nervous system. Protein kinase C and other inflammatory markers present during hyperglycaemia probably also play a role, given hyperglycaemia is a proinflammatory state.

1.11 Thresholds Theory for Cognitive Impairment

It is difficult to predict a single threshold for the onset of cognitive impairment because multiple factors are involved. Satz (1993) developed a 'threshold theory' that comprises three components:

1. Biological threshold for the appearance of cognitive changes once the damage caused by small events such as infarcts exceed the threshold. Several risk factors are implicated in the transition from one state to another; these include APOEe gene carrier status, female gender, low education, smoking, family history of dementia, hypertension, T2DM, and using hormone replacement therapy (Anderson 2014).
2. Principal of additivity: multiple coexisting brain disorders have a cumulative effect.
3. Brain reserve: higher brain reserve can be protective and reduce the likelihood an individual will become cognitively impaired. Lower brain reserve represents vulnerability to cognitive dysfunction.

Brain reserve is a hypothetical construct measured by the number of neurones and the density of interconnections between the neurones, amount of functional brain tissue following damage to the central nervous system, and cognitive processes such as remembering and problem-solving (Stern 2001). However, brain reserve is often operationalised by measuring intelligence or education, which are considered to be surrogate markers of brain reserve.

1.12   Effects of Age and Disease Status on the Way People Learn and Process Information

Research suggests learning and memory skills are largely mediated by the hippocampus and its related limbic and diencephalic systems (Brown and Aggleton 2001). The size of the hippocampus and amygdala begins to decrease at about age 60 and continues to decline with increasing age. The decline in the size of the hippocampus is accompanied by corresponding decline in the ability to learn lists of word pairs and remember stories immediately after hearing them, and after a brief time (immediate recall). A variety of associated diseases affect the hippocampal/limbic systems and their function including hypertension, AGE, and changes in neuronal metabolism and neurotransmitters. Head injuries, chronic alcohol and other toxic substances have a cumulative adverse effect on brain function and exacerbate the adverse effects of hyperglycaemia.

Multiple brain regions are involved in memory. The hippocampus has many functions besides memory: the hippocampus is essential for remembering life episodes, but may not be necessary to retrieve stored information (Squire et al. 2010). The hippocampus is critical for other cognitive tasks in addition to episodic recollection such as the capacity to imagine possible ways in which personal events could have occurred in the past or might occur in the future. It also processes spatial and visual discriminatory tasks and some kinds of linguistic processes. These findings suggest different neurodegenerative disorders have different effects on memory and learning.

Significantly, verbal and memory function are more likely to be affected in people with T2DM aged 60–65 years than other cognitive functions (Ryan and Geckle 2000). Ryan and Geckle (2000) suggested the effects on verbal and memory function are a 'consequence of a synergistic interaction between diabetes-related metabolic derangements and the structural and functional changes occurring in the central nervous system' as the individual ages. Significantly, a growing body of evidence suggest slow cognitive decline:

- Sleeping well
- Eating a healthy diet rich in antioxidants
- Regular exercise
- Avoiding multitasking
- Focusing on the task at hand
- Pursuing intellectual activities 'use it or lose it'.

Memory is not a single process. Memory involves changes at molecular, cellular and synaptic levels and in the neural networks. It involves three stages: encoding, consolidating and retrieving memories. Attending to the information to be encoded, for example, information about GLMs, is important to the way memories are stored. Multitasking is distracting and has detrimental effects on the way memories are consolidated.

Older people with T2DM do not learn as efficiently as their peers without diabetes, and the differences are substantial. Seeing or hearing a series of words and then having to recall the words one at a time in any order appears to be a common deficit (Ryan and Geckle 2000). Diabetes is usually associated with several comorbidities and complications that can affect learning and memory, and these effects are compounded by age-related changes. Significantly, people on insulin perform worse than those on diet and oral glucose lowering medicines (GLM) and also have deficits in abstract reasoning.

Some diabetes self-care tasks involve motor learning. People who can perform motor tasks may do so because their brain recognises previous errors and learns from those errors. The brain controls how much it is prepared to learn from current errors via a process that depends on the person's history of past errors (Herzfeld et al. 2014). It learns more from small errors than large errors.

These issues and changes need to be sensitively and carefully considered and discussed, because some changes such as stopping driving and being admitted to a care home represent significant losses and can be detrimental to an individual's personal dignity (Chap. 2), mental health and autonomy and lead to isolation and depression (Chihuri et al. 2015).

1.13   Management Considerations

Good communication using acceptable language is essential to co-developing personalised care plans (see Chaps. 2 and 3). The impact of language on people with diabetes is described in two position statements (Diabetes Australia 2011; IDF 2014; Dunning et al. 2017; Dickinson et al. 2017). Older people are a highly stigmatised group. Negative ageist attitudes, stereotypes and inappropriate language (baby talk and 'elder speak') are common in the media, society and in health care and affect health professional and 'patient' relationships. Elderspeak leads to resistive behaviours that compound the challenge of communicating with older people with dementias (Herman and Williams 2009).

Importantly, ageist language and attitudes influence treatment decisions and drive the exclusionary research inclusion criteria (www.cib.org.yk/faqs/definitions. aspx). Ageist language also has a significant effect on the self-esteem, confidence and outcomes of older people (Richeson and Shelton 2006).

In addition to being excellent communicators, HPs caring for older people with diabetes need to understand:

- First and foremost, the person who has diabetes and their stories, values, preferences and goals.
- Their own knowledge, attitudes, values and communication skills (Chap. 3).
- Diabetes and its complications and how they affect the individual

- How to assess, manage and monitor diabetes and help them adapt to the change from aiming for near normal blood glucose to a focus on safety and quality of life and using outcome measures relevant to the individual. These may include Patient Reported Outcome Measures (PROMS) but can also be determined by asking the individual.
- The functional and cognitive changes that accompany older age
- The importance of adopting a proactive risk management approach to care that encompasses managing the medicine burden, enhancing independence, accommodating life changes such as planning to stop driving, accepting help and/or admission to a care home.
- When to begin discussing and planning for palliative and end of life care.

As people grow older, the focus on achieving close to normal blood glucose levels to prevent complications is likely to change to a focus on managing complications, promoting comfort and reducing unnecessary treatment burden (Dunning et al. 2013; IDF 2014; Sinclair et al. 2014). Low blood glucose in people aged 75 and older affects cognitive function and quality of life and significantly increases the risk of hypoglycaemia and associated adverse events such as falls, myocardial infarction (Chopra and Kewal 2012) and dementia in the longer term (Yaffe et al. 2013).

Introducing palliative care early in combination with usual care might improve outcomes including nutrition status, physical and cognitive function and life expectancy especially in cancer (World Palliative Care Association (WPCA)/WHO 2014). Regular comprehensive assessments are important to identify functional changes early and modify the care plan when needed.

The individual's functional status and life expectancy need to be considered (Dunning et al. 2010; IDF 2014). Each older person has unique life experiences, genetic characteristics and social circumstances that influence their values, preferences and life goals. HPs must be able to identify and understand an individual's story, identify their values, goals and preferences and the factors that make life worth living for them, to personalise care with them (Chap. 2).

1.14   Blood Glucose Levels

As indicated, there are risks associated with both high and low blood glucose levels in the short term and in the long term. A safe blood glucose range for healthy older people is 5–7 mmol/L: 6–10 mmol/L for those who are frail, and those with dementia and at end of life. Likewise a safe HbA1c range can be >7% up to 8.5% (Dunning et al. 2013; IDF 2014). Generally, blood glucose ranges and HbA1c targets can be higher as the individual grows older, their function and self-care capacity change and their risk of hypoglycaemia increases. However, hyperglycaemia also has adverse effects on cognitive function, increases the risk of infection and ketoacidosis (DKA) in people with T1DM and hyperglycaemic hyperosmolar states (HHS) in people with T2DM (Munshi et al. 2016; Dunning et al. 2013; IDF 2014).

1.15 Hypoglycaemia

Hypoglycaemia is under-recognised, under-reported and under-treated in older people with T1DM and T2DM.

Hypoglycaemia generally refers to blood glucose <3 mmol/L. Hypoglycaemia can be mild if the individual is able to recognise, self-treat and ingest glucose orally. However, mild hypoglycaemia occurs more frequently than people realise and is an aspect of glucose variability as discussed previously.

Hypoglycaemia can be severe and life threatening if the individual is unconscious, requires assistance to manage the episode and requires intravenous glucose because he or she is unable to ingest glucose orally (Anderson et al. 2014). Continuous glucose monitoring (CGM) shows people have many mild unrecognised episodes of hyperglycaemia and these episodes contribute to severe hypoglycaemia.

Hypoglycaemia is common in older people with T1DM and T2DM and often not recognised due to changed symptoms that occur with age and long duration of diabetes. Hypoglycaemia has a negative impact on well-being, lifestyle and safety. Neuroglycopaenic symptoms such as confusion and behaviour change are more common than the well-known adrenergic symptoms: sweating, palpitations and anxiety in older people, because of the effect of low blood glucose on the neurones in the brain (Cryer 2007).

The counter-regulatory hormone response to falling blood glucose such as glucagon that liberate glucose stores when blood glucose is low diminish with long duration of diabetes, but can be lost early in the course of T1DM (Siafarikas et al. 2012). These changes can affect the individual's ability to recognise and self-manage hypoglycaemia. They highlight the need for each individual with diabetes to have a personalised hypoglycaemia risk assessment and care plan that encompasses:

- Safe blood glucose range based on their personal diabetes risk
- Safe HbA1c range
- Blood glucose testing regimen that suits their glucose lowering medicine action profiles; insulin and sulphonylureas are associated with high hypoglycaemia risk especially if the person has compromised renal function (Heald et al. 2017) (Chap. 6) and those with long duration of diabetes (Hope et al. 2017).
- Education for family and other carers.

Early recognition of hypoglycaemia and treatment are essential (Kenny 2013). Hypothermia can occur during severe hypoglycaemic episodes in cold weather and impede recovery. Hypoglycaemia is also associated with falls risk and injuries such as fractures and head injuries and affects driving safety. It is important to realise that motorised wheel chairs and some farm equipment also pose a safety risk.

Risk factors for hypoglycaemia in older people are described in hypoglycaemia risk assessment tools such as the one in the McKellar Guidelines (Dunning et al. 2013, reproduced with permission) and The Edinburgh Hypoglycaemia Scale (Graveling et al. 2013). The presence of any one of these factors represents high risk of hypoglycaemia for older people. The more risk factors present, the great the risk. The individual's hypoglycaemia risk factors can be decided by discussing the factors with them and/or their families.

The hypoglycaemia care plan should be based on the risk assessment and might include:

- Everybody associated with the older person being 'hypo aware' without being intrusive
- Helping the individual and carers recognise atypical signs of hypoglycaemia; for example, learning to recognise the individual personal body cues through programmes such as Blood Glucose Awareness Training Program (Cox et al. 2001).
- Ways to manage hypoglycaemic episodes
- Ensuring in-date glucagon is available to treat severe hypoglycaemia and is replaced as soon as it is used
- Undertaking medicine reviews, avoiding medicines that contribute to hypoglycaemia or using such medicines in the lowest effective dose, and asking about glucose lowering complementary medicines use
- Assessing renal function regularly
- Considering the action profile of glucose lowering medicines and planning meals and blood glucose monitoring frequency and activity to match the action profile.

1.16 Hyperglycaemia

'Safe' blood glucose and HbA1c ranges were described earlier in the chapter. Many factors, besides blood glucose, can affect HbA1c and these need to be considered when deciding treatment (Dunning and Cukier 2014). These include anaemia, which is common in older people, haemoglobinopathies and bleeding. Likewise, HbA1c is an average measure of blood glucose over the past 3 months and does not reflect glucose variability (Lipska and Krumholtz 2017).

Hyperglycaemia can be a consequence of intercurrent illness such as urinary tract infections, infected foot ulcers and respiratory disease. Older people need a personalised 'sick' day care plan to help them manage such illnesses to help them stay out of hospital, if possible. However hyperglycaemia affects cognitive function and contributes to incontinence and dehydration, which predisposed them to HHS and DKA which usually require a hospital admission.

Correction/top up insulin doses are often used to treat isolated episodes of hyperglycaemia in aged care homes: *they should not be used* (Cheung and Chipps 2010; American Geriatric Society 2015). Top up insulin doses lead to an adverse cycle of hypoglycaemia and rebound hyperglycaemia. However, older people using an insulin pump or basal bolus insulin may use correction doses with meals to cover the carbohydrate load or to manage sick days. Older people are at risk of infections and preventative care such as vaccinations should be considered (McGovern et al. 2016).

Educating the individual and family carers, collaboratively developing a personalised plan for managing intercurrent illnesses (sick day care plan) and reviewing and adjusting medicine doses, when indicated are key nursing care strategies to manage hyperglycaemia.

Delirium is characterised by changes in attention, awareness and cognition and is associated with adverse outcomes and increased mortality in older people. It can be a consequence of hyperglycaemia. It occurs in 1 in 5 older people, 33% of people who have surgery and 80% older people in intensive care (Frick et al. 2002). Significantly, medicines are implicated in 22–89% of people with delirium. Nurses can use the Confusion Assessment Method to help identify delirium (Wei et al. 2008).

1.17 Preventive Health Care

Preventive health care should be included in holistic personalised care plans for older people with diabetes. Preventative health care includes relevant immunisation, e.g. pneumonia, influenza and zostervax, relevant health screening such a mammograms and bowel and prostate checks, oral health and hearing assessments, and assessing functional status and self-care activities and driving (Dunning 2016).

It is important to assess quality of life regularly. Standardised, valid tools such as the Wellbeing Index can be used, but in keeping with personalised care, it is more useful to ask the person to describe three to five things that make life meaningful for them and regularly ask about any changes in these issues. Likert scales can be developed to quantify changes. These are known as patient-generated tools (Jenkinson and McGee 1998) and are more likely to reflect issues relevant to the individual.

1.18 Pets and Companion Animals

Pets and companion animals, especially dogs and cats, are essential life companions to many older people: sometimes pets are the only family with whom the person has a meaningful relationship. Significantly, many people, including the author, regard pets as members of the family (Crist 2017). Some companion animals provide essential help for people with diabetes, for example, guide dogs for vision impaired people and some animals warn their owners about low blood glucose and impending seizures.

The health and social benefits of pets and companion animals are well documented in care homes and end of life care settings and when a partner dies (International Federation on Ageing (IFA) undated).

Older people become very concerned for their pet's welfare during illness and when they find it functionally difficult to care from their pets. They often prioritise their pet's welfare over their own. Not being able to take beloved pets into a care facility can be particularly stressful and lead to grief, withdrawal and depression, even when the home allows visiting animals.

Likewise, many pet owners assume a significant carer burden caring for sick and frail older pets and significant grief when a pet dies (Crist 2017). The study highlights the complexity of human-animal relationships and the importance of taking such relationships seriously when working with older people generally and those with diabetes.

1.19 Family Carers

Family carers provide a significant amount of unpaid care: >60% of the care is provided by a spouse who often has health care problems including diabetes. Health status influences family cares' decision to admit their loved one to a care facility (Family Caregiver Alliance 2010). Family carers undertake over 10.1 h of care/week for people on oral glucose lowering medicines and 14.1 h/week when the person is on insulin compared to 6 h/week caring for people without diabetes (Langa et al. 2002).

Carers are at risk of stress-related illnesses such as intercurrent infections, cardiovascular events and dying during their time providing care and in the weeks and months following bereavement (Mostofsky et al. 2012; Carey et al. 2014). In turn, carer ill health and depression affect well-being and quality of life of the person they care for (Kitzelman 2016). Therefore, carers also need a care plan and their care needs to be monitored as carefully as the older person with diabetes. They often require education about taking on diabetes self-care tasks and managing hypo- and hyperglycaemia. Older carers also need preventative health care such as vaccinations and relevant screening.

1.20 Nutrition, Activity, Sarcopenia and Frailty

Eating a healthy diet high in fruit and vegetables and nuts, reducing salt intake, limiting alcohol, keeping active and stopping smoking are important (see Chap. 5). Malnutrition is common in older people and compromises independence, increases hypoglycaemia risk, contributes to deficiency disorders such as anaemia and vitamins C, D and B_{12}. Some older people require nutrition supplements.

Nutrition is an important part of an holistic assessment to determine whether supplements are indicated. HPs can refer the individual to a dietitian and/or a speech therapist if the person has swallowing difficulties, for advice. Malnutrition increases the risk of intercurrent infections, which often result in hyperglycaemia, and oral health problems, which compromise food intake and enjoyment, can contribute to medicine-related adverse events (Do-Yeon et al. 2016). Malnutrition is associated with increased morbidity.

Subcutaneous fat decreases and visceral fat increases with increasing age and may contribute to reduced insulin sensitivity. Muscle mass reduces by 1–2% annually after age 30, 1.5–3% after age 60 and at a faster rate after age 75 (Sinclair et al. 2017). Consequently, functional impairments can be present in middle age and may continue to decline over the next 10 years (Brown et al. 2017).

Loss of muscle mass, sarcopenia, is common in people with diabetes (Fiatarone Singh 2010; Jang 2016). Sarcopenia and diabetes appear to have a bidirectional relationship: sarcopenia contributes toT2DM and diabetes exacerbates the progression to sarcopenia and frailty (Sinclair et al. 2017). Insulin protects protein synthesis in muscle in young people and helps conserve muscle mass, but not in older people (Scott et al. 2016).

Sarcopenia predisposes the individual to frailty, which occurs in >11% of people age 65 and older (Abdelhafz et al. 2015). Overweight individuals can be frail because of low muscle mass (sarcopenic obesity). Weight loss in such individual's might exacerbate frailty risks such as under-nutrition, falls and hypoglycaemia. Frailty can be assessed using various valid 'frailty scales' as part of an holistic assessment to plan care. However, the scales measure various aspects of frailty and HPs need to understand what they measure to use them effectively. Examples include The Frail Scale (Rockwood et al. 2005).

Being active is important to overall health but must be relevant to the individual's interest and functional status. Walking, swimming, dancing, Tai chi and yoga can be beneficial for physical and mental health. In addition, Tai chi improves balance and flexibility and reduces falls risk (Kuramoto 2006; Do-Yeon et al. 2016). Tai chi (exercise and mind care) helps maintain mobility and psychological well-being, reduces fear of falling and improves sleep and cardiac function (Kuramoto 2006). Progressive strength training and adequate protein in the diet help preserve muscle mass and have positive effects on cognition especially, when strength training commences before old age (Fiatarone Singh 2010).

1.21 Mental Health, Cognitive Function and Dementia

Hypo- and hyperglycaemia can affect cognitive function in the short and longer term. HPs should plan to undertake heath assessments and provide education when the individual's blood glucose is in an appropriate range.

T2DM is associated with dementia (Yaffe et al. 2013), which often presents with behaviour changes and is challenging and stressful for HPs and family carers (Chap. 8). People with dementia prescribed insulin might need dose and a dose regimen centred around when they eat to reduce hypoglycaemia risk; thus a flexible approach managing medicines and diet that focus on safety might be needed. People with dementia are at high risk of under-recognised and under-treated pain and depression and suicide (Ibrahim et al. 2017). Risk factors for depression include:

- High HbA1c
- Under/untreated insomnia
- Pain
- Vascular disease
- Significant losses and grief such as loss of function and independence
- Death of a partner or beloved pet
- Social isolation

- Nutritional deficiency
- Some medicines
- Alcohol
- Living with the burden of diabetes and its associated medicine and care burdens for long periods of time.

Blood glucose monitoring can also be challenging but is important in people with dementia on insulin and sulphonylureas because of the high hypoglycaemia risk and difficulty the individual, family identifying hypoglycaemia in people with cognitive changes. Continuous glucose monitoring can be helpful but is expensive and there are practical issues such as the person removing the glucose sensors. Medicines can also contribute to confusion and behaviour change.

1.22 Planning for Palliative and End of Life Care

Public health policies and medicines do not offer eternal life. They do offer a longer more comfortable life to many people and a reasonable chance of premature death in many countries but most people die before age 100.

The following Japanese death poem highlights the inevitability of death. It is the death poem of the Zen Buddhist monk Toko. He was commenting on the pretentiousness of some other author's death poems. Toko broke with tradition by explicitly mentioning death: the tradition was to use metaphors for death such as falling leaves. Death is still inevitable and we still hide behind euphemisms and less poetic metaphors such as 'passed on' and 'gone'.

Death poems
Are mere delusion -
Death is death. (Toko 1710–1795 at age 85)

The importance of planning for end of life care re-emerged in the past 5 years and is increasingly viewed as a viable choice rather than as treatment (or health professional) failure. Most people died in their homes in 'the olden days' not in hospitals, intensive care units (ICU) or aged care homes. Modern research shows people still want to die in their own homes, but <10% actually do die at home or in their place of choice (Sweirssen and Duckett 2014; World Palliative Care Association (WPCA)/World Health Organisation (WHO) 2014).

Palliative care can be implemented with usual diabetes care to manage unpleasant symptoms that arise from diabetes complications and/or other diseases such as cancer. Palliative care can include surgery to improve distressing symptoms. Palliative care improves quality of life and often life expectancy (WPCA/WHO 2014) and can ease the transition to end of life care. Helping older people with diabetes and families plan for the end of life is important.

HPs can use tools The Gold Standards Framework (2011) and Guidelines for Managing Diabetes at the end of Life (Dunning et al. 2010) to initiate discussions about the person's values, goals and preferences and to document them in Advance Care Directives, depending on the culture and the legal system of the relevant country.

1.23 Summary

Caring for older people is a privilege. It can be challenging, very rewarding and often sad. Older people with diabetes are unique individuals and their care must be designed with them where possible. Care must suit their individual needs, values and preferences and be regularly reassessed. It must include planning for end of life care. Care is often delivered by family members. They must be educated and supported. In hospitals, care homes and other care settings care must be delivered by appropriately educated, compassionate health professionals.

1.24 Reflection Points

Mrs. Blogs has early dementia. She is 79 and has lived with T2DM for 30 years. She has neuropathic foot disease and used a walking stick because: *'I stumble a bit sometimes'*. She is on long-acting insulin at night and rapid-acting insulin before each meal: *'I find that a bit of a problem because I do not have much appetite these days'*. She enjoys walking her dog. Her husband is 82 and provides care such as assistance with some ADLs and IADLs.

Mr. Blogs recently had a hip replacement: *'it's OK now but I have to have the other one done sometime and I am worried about how she will cope. She tripped over the other day and had trouble getting up'*.

1. What more information do you need to develop a care plan for Mrs. Blogs?
2. Does Mr. Blogs need a care plan too?
3. Will one care plan be appropriate for both of them?
4. What are the key risks for each person and the dog?
5. What forward planning needs to be considered?

References

Abdelhafz A, Rodrigeuz-Manas L, Morley J, Sinclair A (2015) Hypoglycaemia in older people- a less well recognised risk factor for frailty. Ageing Dis 6:156–167

American Geriatric Society (2015) Identifying medicines that should be avoided in older people or used with caution. Updated BEERs criteria. www.americangeriatrics.org/.../beers/BeersCriteria

Anderson P (2014) Managing diabetes in nursing and care homes. Nurs Times 110(34/35):20–22

Anderson M, Powell J, Campbell K et al (2014) Optimal management of type 2 diabetes in patients at increased risk of hypoglycaemia. Diabetes Metab Syndr Obes 7:85–94

Ari Y, Martin-Ruiz C, Takayama M et al (2015) Inflammation, but not telomere length predicts successful ageing at extreme old age: a longitudinal study of semi-supercentenarians. EBioMedicine 2:1549–1558

Australian Centre for Social Innovation (tasci) (2016)

Australian Medicines Handbook (2017) https://shop.amh.net.au/products/books/2017

Brown M, Aggleton J (2001) Recognition memory: what are the roles of the perirhinal cortex and hippocampus? Nat Rev Neurosci 2:51–61

Brown R, Diaz-Ramirez Z, Boscardin W et al (2017) Functional impairment in middle age: a cohort study. Ann Intern Med. https://doi.org/10.7326/m17-0496

Butler R (1969) Age-ism: another form of bigotry. The Gerontologist 9(4, Part 1):243–246

Butler R (1980) Ageism: a foreword. J Soc Issues 36(2):8–11

Callahan M (2015) Searching for Grace Kelly. Mariner Books, New York

Carey M, Shah S, DeWilde S et al (2014) Increased risk of acute cardiovascular events after partner bereavement. JAMA Intern Med. https://doi.org/10.1001/jamainternalmed.2013.14558

Cheung N, Chipps R (2010) Sliding scale insulin: will the false idol finally fall? Intern Med J 40:662–664

Chihuri S, Mielenz T, DiMaggio C, Betz M, DiGuiseppi C, Jones V, Guohua L (2015) driving cessation and health outcomes in older adults foundation for traffic safety. https://www.aaafoundation.org/sites/.../DrivingCessationReport.pdf

Chopra S, Kewal A (2012) Does hypoglycaemia cause hypoglycaemic events? Indian J Endocrinol Metab 10(1):102–104

Cox D, Goner-Frederick L, Polonsky W et al (2001) Blood Glucose Awareness training (BGAT-2). Diabetes Care 24(4):637–642

Crist C (2017) 'Caregiver burden' affects people with sick pets too. http://bit.ly2wRYidw

Cryer P (2007) Hypoglycaemia, functional brain failure and brain death. J Clin Investig 117(4):866–870

Debrabant B, Sorensen M, Flachsbart F et al (2014) Human longevity and variation in DNA damage response and repair: a study of the contribution of sub-processes using competitive geneset analysis. Eur J Hum Genet 22(9):1131–1136

Diabetes Australia (2011) A new language for diabetes: position statement. mail@diabetesvic.org.au

Dickinson J, Guzman S, Marynuik M et al (2017) The use of language in diabetes care and education. Diabetes Care 40(12):1790–1799

Do-Yeon K, Chang-O K, Hyunjung L (2016) Quality of diet and level of physical performance related to inflammatory markers in community-dwelling frail elderly people. J Nutr. https://doi.org/10.1016/j.mut.2016.12.023

Dunning T (2016) Assessing older people with diabetes in Australia. Diabetes Prim Care Aust 1(4):1–6

Dunning T (2017) Ancient wisdom, modern science—do the twain meet? World Diabetes Day Professorial Lecture, Geelong, VIC

Dunning T, Cukier K (2014) HbA1c: chasing numbers or considering context? J Diabetes Nurs 18(1):13–18

Dunning T, Sinclair S (2014) Glucose lowering medicines and older people with diabetes: the importance of comprehensive assessments and pharmacovigilance. Nurs Care 3(3). https://doi.org/10.4172/2167-1168.1000160

Dunning T, Savage S, Duggn N (2010) Guidelines for managing diabetes at the end of life. https://www.adma.org.au/.../35-guidelines-for-managing-diabetes-at-the-end-of-life.html

Dunning T, Savage S, Duggan N. (2013) The McKellar guidelines for managing older people with diabetes in residential and other care settings. http://www.adma.org.au/clearinghouse/doc_details/133-the-mckellar-guidelines-for-managing-older-people-with-diabetes-in-residential-and-other-care-settings_9dec2013.html

Dunning T, Speight J, Bennett C (2017) Language, the 'diabetes restricted cade/dialect' and what it means for people with diabetes and clinicians. Diabetes Educ 43(1):18–26

Family Caregiver Alliance (2010) Caregiver health: a population at risk. http://www.caregiver.org/caregiver/jsp/content_node.jsp?nodeid=1822. Accessed June 2016

Fiatarone Singh M (2010) Exercise comes of age as medicine for older adults. Res Dig 10(3):1–13

Foster S (2017) High-risk foot and the effect of deteriorating reneal function and dialysis in people with diabetes. J Diabetes Nurs 21(1):10–18

Frick D, Agostini I, Inouye S (2002) Delirium superimposed on dementia: a systematic review. J Am Geriatr Soc 124:165–183

Genova L (2009) Still Alice. Simon & Schuster, London

Gold Standards Framework Centre (2011) Prognostic indicator guidance. http://www.goldstandardsframework.org.uk/cd-content/uploads/files/General%Files/Prognostic%20Indicator%20Guidance%20October%201011.pdf

Graveling A, Deary I, Frier B (2013) Acute hypoglycaemia impairs executive cognitive function in adults with and without type 1 diabetes. Diabetes Care 36(10):3240–3246. https://doi.org/10.2337/dc13-0194

Hambling C, Seidu S, Davies MJ et al (2016) Older people with type 2 diabetes, including those with chronic kidney disease or dementia, are commonly overtreated with sulfonylurea or insulin therapies. Diabet Med. https://doi.org/10.1111/dme.133380

Heald A, Anderson S, Cortes G, et al (2017) Hypoglycaemia in the over 75s: understanding the predisposing factors in type 2 diabetes (T2DM). Prim Care Diabetes. https://doi.org/10.1016/j.pcd.2017.08.002

Herman R, Williams K (2009) Elderspeak's influence on resistiveness to care: focus on behavioural events. Am J Alzheimer's Dis Other Demen 24(5):417–423

Herzfeld D, Vaswami P, Marko M, Shadmehr R (2014) A memory of errors in semsorimotor learning. Science 345(6203):1349–1353

Holstein (2006) 317(46). http://www.lco-cdo.org/en/older-adults-lco-funded-papers-charmaine-spencer-sectionII

Hope S, Taylor P, Shields B, et al (2017) Are we missing hypoglycaemia? Elderly patients with insulin-treated diabetes present to primary care frequently with non-specific symptoms associated with hypoglycaemia. Prim Care Diabetes. https://doi.org/10.1016/j.pcd.2017.08.0004

Horvath S (2013) DNA methylation age of human tissues and cell types. Genome Biol 14(10):R115

Hubbard B, Sinclair D (2014) Small molecule SIRT1 activators for the treatment of ageing and age related diseases. Trends Pharmacol Sci 25(3):146–154

Ibrahim J, Bugeja L, Willoughby M, Bevan M, Kipsaina C, Young C, Pham T, Ranson D (2017) Premature deaths of nursing home residents: an epidemiological analysis. Med J Aust. https://doi.org/10.5694/mja16.00873

IDF (2014) Language philosophy technical document and recommendations for communicating with and about people with diabetes www.idf.org

International Diabetes Federation (IDF) (2013) Global guidelines for managing older people with type 2 diabetes. www.idf.org

International Federation on Ageing (IFA) (undated) Measuring the benefits: companion animals and the health of older persons. ifa-fiv.org

Jang H (2016) Society, family and diabetes and older adults. Diabetes Metab 40:182–189

Jenkinson C, McGee H (1998)Health status measurement Radcliffe Medical Press, Oxford

Jumnila R, List E, Berryman D et al (2013) The GH/IGF-1 axis in ageing and longevity. Nat Rev Endocrinol 9(6):366–376

Karlsson F, Tremaroli V, Nookaew L (2013) Gut metagenome in European women with normal, impaired and diabetic glucose control. Nature 489:99–103

Kenny C (2013) When hypoglycaemia is not obvious: diagnosing and treating under-recognised and undisclosed hypoglycaemia. Prim Care Diabetes. http://dx.doi.org/10.1016.j.pcd.09.002

King K, Peacock J, Donnelly R (1999) The UK prospective diabetes study (UKPDS): clinical and therapeutic implications for type 2 diabetes. Br J Clin Pharmacol 48(5):643–646

Kirkman S, Briscoe V, Clark N et al (2012) Diabetes in older adults. Diabetes Care 35:2650–2664

Kitzelman K (2016) How does carer wellbeing relate to perceived quality of life in patients with cancer? J Clin Oncol. https://doi.org/10.1200/oco.2016.67.343

Kovalchev B, Cobelli C (2016) Glucose variability: timing. Risk, analysis and relationship to hypoglycaemia in diabetes. Diabetes Care 39:502–510

Kuramoto A (2006) Therapeutic benefits of tai chi exercise: research review. Wis Med J 105(7):42–46

Langa K, Vijans S, Hayward R et al (2002) Informal caregiving for diabetes and non-diabetic compilations among elderly Americans. J Gerontol Psychiatry Sci 57:S177–S186

Lansky D (1998) Measuring what matters to the public. Health Aff 17(4):40–41

Launer L, Miller M, Williamson J et al (2011) Effects of randomisation to intensive glucose lowering on brain structure and function in type 2 diabetes ACCORD Memory in Diabetes Study. Lancet Neurol 10(11):969–977

Lipska K, Krumholtz H (2017) Is haemoglobin A1c the right outcome for studies of diabetes? J Am Med Assoc. http://jamanetwork.com/pdfaccess.ashx?url=data/journals/jama/o/on01/26/2017

Lopez-Otin C, Partridge L, Serrano M, Kromer G (2013) Hallmarkes of ageing. Cell 153:1194–1216

Mc Fadden S, Thibault J (2001) *Chronos to Kairos* Christian perspectives in time and ageing. In: McFadden S, Atchley R (eds) Aging and the meaning of time. Springer Publishing Company, New York, pp 229–250

McCall A (1992) The impact of diabetes on the CNS. Diabetes 41(5):557–570

McCoy R, Lopska K, Yao X et al (2016) Intensive treatment and severe hypoglycaemia among adults with type 2 diabetes. J Am Med Assoc Intern Med 176:969–978

McGovern A, Hine J, de Lausignan S (2016) Infection risk in elderly people with reduced glycaemic control. Lancet Diab Endocrinol 4:303–304

Meneilly G. (2011) Diabetes in the elderly. Canadian Journal Diabetes, June 13–14

Mostofsky E, Maclure M,Sherwood J (2012) Risk of acute myocardial infarction after death of a significant person in one's life: the determinant of MI study. Circulation. http://circ.ahajournals.org/content/early/1012/o1/09/CIRCULATIONaha.111.061770

Munshi M, Florez H, Huang E et al (2016) Management of diabetes in long-term care and skilled nursing facilities: a position statement of the American Diabetes Association. Diabetes Care 39(2):308–318

Nathan D and for the DCCT/EDIC Research Group (2014) The diabetes control and complications trial/epidemiology of diabetes interventions and complications study at 30 years: overview. Diabetes Care 37(1):9–16. https://doi.org/10.2337/dc13-2112

National Ageing Research Institute (NARI) (2017) The New Middle Age: ways to thrive in the longevity economy

National Institute of Clinical Excellence (2002) (NICE) (2015) Diabetes in Adults: management (NG28) NICE London. www.nice.org.uk/Guidance/NG28. Accessed June 2017

Nelson P, Carnegie P, Martin J et al (2003) Demystified human endogenous retroviruses. J Clin Pathol 56(1):11–16

Ogurtsova K, da Rocha FJ, Huang Y et al (2017) IDF Diabetes Atlas: global estimates for the prevalence of diabetes for 2015–2040. Diabetes Res Clin Pract 128:40–50

Passarino G, De Ranao F, Montesantto A (2016) Human longevity: genetics or Lifestyle? It takes two to tango. Immun Ageing. https://doi.org/10.1180/s12979-016-0066-z

Peters K, Davis W, Ito J et al (2017) Identification of novel circulating biomarkers predicting rapid decline in renal function in type 2 diabetes: the fremantle diabetes study phase II. Diabetes Care 40(11):1548–1555

Petersen K, Dufour S, Befroy D et al (2004) Impaired mitochondrial activity in the insulin-resistant offspring of patients with type 2 diabetes. N Engl J Med 350:664–671

Raule N, Sevini F, Li S et al (2016) The co-occurrence of mDNA mutations on different oxidative phosphorylation subunits not detected by haplogroup analysis affects human longevity and is population specific. Ageing Cell 13(3):401–407

Richeson J, Shelton N (2006) A social psychological perspective on stigmatisation of older adults National Library of Medicine. https://www.ncbi.nih.gov/books/NBK83758/

Rizzo M, Marfella R, Barberi M et al (2010) Relationships between daily acute glucose fluctuations and cognitive performance among aged type 2 diabetic patients. Diabetes Care 33(10):2169–2174

Rockwood K, Song A, MacKnight C et al (2005) A global clinical measure of fitness and frailty in elderly people. Can Med Assoc J 173:489–495

Ryan C, Geckle M (2000) Why is learning and memory dysfunction in type 2 diabetes limited to older adults? Diabetes Metab Res Rev 16(5):308–315

Satz P (1993) Brain reserve capacity on symptom onset after brain injury: a formulation and review of evidence for threshold theory. Neuropsychology 7:273–295

Scarletti J, Schwartz M (2015) Gut-brain mechanisms controlling glucose homeostasis. F1000Prime Rep 7:12. https://doi.org/10.12703/P7-12

Schachter F, Faure-Deland L, Geunot F et al (1994) Genetic associations with human longevity at APOE and ACE Loci. Nat Genet 6(1):29–32

Scott D, deCourten B, Ebeling P (2016) Sarcopaenia: a potential cause and consequence of type 2 diabetes in Australian. Med J Aust 205(7):329–333

Siafarikas A, Johnston R, Bulsara M et al (2012) Early loss of the glucagon response to hypoglycemia in adolescents with type 1 diabetes. Diabetes Care 35(8):1757–1762. https://doi.org/10.2337/dc11-2010

Sinclair A, Gadsby R, Penfold S, Croxson S, Bayer A (2001) Prevalence of diabetes in care home residents. Diabetes Care 24(6):1066–1068

Sinclair A, Dunning T, Rodrigeuz-Manas L (2014) Diabetes in older people: new insights and remaining challenges. Lancet Diab Endocrinol. https://doi.org/10.1016/s2213

Sinclair A, Abdelhafiz A, Rodrigeuz-Manas L (2017) Frailty and sarcopenia—newly emerging and high impact complications of diabetes. J Diabetes Complicat 31:1465–1473

Sorensen M, Thinggaard M, Nygaard M et al (2012) Genetic variation in TERT and TERC and human leucocyte telomere length and longevity: a cross-sectional and longitudinal analysis. Ageing Cell 11(2):223–227

Squire L, van der Horst A, McDuff S et al (2010) Role of the hippocampus in remembering the past and imagining the future. Proc Natl Acad Sci U S A 107(44):19044–19048. https://doi.org/10.1073/pnas.1014391107

Stern Y (2001) What is cognitive reserves? Theory and research application of the reserve concept. J Int Neuropsychol Soc 8:448–460

Sun X, Walker N, Wagner M, Bachman D (2012) APOE genotype in the diagnosis of Alzheimer's disease in patients with cognitive impairment. J Alzheimer's Dis Other Demen 27(5):15–20

Swerissen H, Duckett, S (2014) Dying well. Grattan Institute. ISBN: 978-1-925015-61-4. https://grattan.edu.au/wp-content/uploads/2014/09/815-dying-well.pdf

The Diabetes Control and Complications Trial (DCCT) Research Group (1993) The effect of intensive treatment of diabetes on the development and progression of long-term complications in insulin-dependent diabetes mellitus. N Engl J Med 329:977–986. PMID: 8366922

Turner R, Stratton I, Horton V, Manley S, Zimmet P, Mackay IR, Shattock M, Bottazzo GF, Holman R, UKPDS 25 (1997) Autoantibodies to islet-cell cytoplasm and glutamic acid decarboxylase for prediction of insulin requirement in type 2 diabetes. Lancet 350:1288–1293

United Kingdom Prospective Diabetes Study (UKPDS) Prospective Diabetes Study Group (1998) Intensive blood glucose control with sulphonylureas or insulin compared with conventional treatment and risk of complications in patients with type 2 diabetes. UKPDS 33. Lancet 352:837–853

Wagner W (2017) Epgenetics, ageing clocks in mice and men. Genome Biol 18:107. https://doi.org/10.1186/s.13059-017-1245-8

Wei L, Fearing M, Sternberg E, Inouye S (2008) The Confusion Assessment Method (CAM): a systematic review of current usage. J Am Geriatr Soc 56(5):823–830. doi: https://doi.org/10.1111/j.1532-5415.2008.01674.x. Accessed April 2017

Weng S, Landes S (2017) Culture and language discordance in the workplace: evidence form the national home aide health survey. The Gerontologist 57(5):900–909

World Health Organisation (WHO) (2002) Proposed working definition of an older person in Africa for the MDS Project. Accessed April 2017

WHO (2017) definition of palliative care WHO. www.who.int/cancer/palliative/definition/en/

Worldwide Palliative Care Alliance (WPCA)/World Health Organisation (WHO) (2014) www.THEWPCA.org. Accessed April 2017

Yaffe C, Fulvey C, Hamilton M (2013) Association between hypoglycaemia and dementia in a biracial cohort of older adults with diabetes mellitus. JAMA Intern Med 173(14):1300–1306

Yaffe K, Vittinghoff E, Pletcher M et al (2014) Early adult to midlife cardiovascular risk and cognitive decline. Circulation 129(15):1560–1567

Zanh J, Kaplan M, Fischer S et al (2015) Expansion of a novel endogenous retrovirus throughout the pericentromeres of modern humans. Genome Biol 16(1):74–92

The Art of Shared Decision-Making and Personalising Care with Older People with Diabetes

2

Trisha Dunning

> *Dr. Williams discussing patients seen that day with Nina, a medical student, said:*
>
> *Let's see, we saw three kids today with the same disease, middle ear infection.*
>
> *Nina: But from such different families!*
>
> *Dr. Williams: Oh, Yeah, you can take the same germ, give it to three different families and come up with three different problems that you treat in three different ways. The illness equals the disease and the person.*
>
> *Nina: What a revolutionary idea to treat the patient first and the disease second.*
>
> *Dr. Williams: …what is really revolutionary is to treat the person and the disease at the same time.*
>
> *(Karr undated)*

Key Points

- Personalised care is as essential to safe quality care and optimal outcomes as evidence-based care.
- Personalising care is an art that involves active listening, being mindful, being able to interpret people's stories and using the information to create care plans *with* them.
- Words are powerful. Select them carefully and use them wisely.
- Language must be congruent with the philosophy of personalised care.

T. Dunning, A.M., M.Ed., Ph.D., R.N., C.D.E.
Centre for Quality and Patient Safety Research, Barwon Health Partnership, Deakin University, Geelong, VIC, Australia
e-mail: trisha.dunning@barwonhealth.org.au;
trisha.dunning@deakin.edu.au

29

2.1   Introduction

Modern health care is influenced by two main concepts: personalised care and evidence-based care (Bensing 2000). Both concepts influence the clinical decision-making process. Both are highly relevant, but different, aspects of care: the first as old as time, the second relatively new. Bridging the gap between the two philosophies is essential to ensure the art or human aspect informs and is informed by evidence. Evidence-based medicine/care enables individual health professionals (HP) to integrate their clinical experience and knowledge with scientific evidence. Such evidence is largely disease oriented and derived from randomised control trials, which are not person-centred per se, but can be used to deliver personalised care, see Chap. 4.

Qualitative methods are more likely to elicit information relevant to the person with the disease and can add a person-centred perspective to evidence-based recommendations. Significantly, Glas (1996) stated that physicians should never neglect psychosocial issues or the uniqueness of the individual when using the best available evidence. In addition, people are more satisfied when HPs consider the non-medical aspects of their illnesses and treat them as a person (Frederikson 1995). Conversely, people are less satisfied when HPs explore psychosocial factors when the individual only wants to discuss the biomedical aspects of their disease (Frederikson 1995). Frederikson's findings highlight the fact that good communication is essential to establish a common agenda for consultations and education and requires active listening, empathy and the ability to find the meaning in the individual's personal story, see Chap. 3.

I give an annual professorial lecture on the closest Friday to World Diabetes Day (November 14th) every year. The lectures are designed to be scholarly, but also to challenge, to entertain and are an avenue to advocate for older people with diabetes. My lecture in 2016 was entitled: *Personalised diabetes care: myth, mantra or reality?* This chapter is largely based on that lecture. The lecture was based on a review of the literature, personal experience, and stories and discussions with older people with diabetes.

2.2   What Is Personalised Care?

Personalised care is one of the most important determinants of health outcomes (Richardson et al. 2001). It is associated with improved health outcomes, improved survival time, satisfaction, well-being and reduced costs (Rathert et al. 2013). There is also moderate quality evidence that personalised care is associated with small reductions in HbA1c, depression and self-efficacy but not on body mass index, LDL cholesterol, diastolic blood pressure or the physical or mental components of subjective health status using SF-36 or SF-12 (Coulter et al. 2015).

Personalised care is a multidimensional concept and is difficult to operationalise in measurable elements (Bensing 2000). There is no agreed definition but there is agreement about the core principles that underpin the concept: respect, dignity, self-efficacy, empowerment, and finding meaning and purpose (spirituality), enabling therapeutic partnerships based on equality.

A range of terms are used to refer to personalised care in the literature, including patient-centred, patient-oriented, individualised, tailored, person-centred, consumer-centred, person-focused, customer-focused, client oriented, communication-centred and resident-centred. The plethora of terms gives rise to a series of questions:

- Are 'we' all talking about the same thing but actually mean something different?
- Do these terms mean the same thing?
- Do they mean the same thing to everybody?
- Are they congruent with the philosophy of personalised care?
- Should 'somebody' select a term, implement it, and then use it consistently?

Starfield (2011) suggested patient-centred and person-focused are different in that patient-centred is 'visit-based' whereas person-focused is based on the 'accumulated knowledge of people' and focuses on the whole person. However, 'accumulated knowledge of people is ambiguous and it is not clear whose knowledge Starfield was referring to; the individual and their HPs or both. David Strain in Chap. 10 distinguishes between personalised and individualised care.

I choose to use 'personalised care' because it contains the word 'person'. It is imperative to know the person who has the disease (diabetes), their explanatory models for health and ill health, their reasons for consulting HPs and their values, preferences and goals to develop personalised care plans. Likewise, the term reflects the ethical and moral responsibility HPs have to treat every person with respect, to support their autonomy, and is inclusive.

You will note the title of the book refers to personalising care *with* older people with diabetes, not *for* people with diabetes and includes shared decision-making. When I submitted the book proposal to the Commissioning editor, she asked:

Should the title read '…personalisng care **for** older people with diabetes?'

Grammatically that is correct; however it suggests doing things to or for people rather than **with** them. Thus, it does not encompass key aspects of personalised care such as the importance of the individual in the process, shared decision-making and therapeutic relationships. I was very pleased when she accepted the explanation for the proposed title.

Several definitions of personalised are described in Box 2.1. Other definitions include the following:

'Respectful of and responsive to individual patient preferences, needs, and values, and ensuring the patient values guide all clinical decisions' (Richardson et al. 2001). Richardson et al. refer to an individual's values, preferences and needs, which are important aspects of personalising care. They allude to shared decision-making then use the word 'patient', which to me suggests a hierarchy, however well intended. Communication is essential to eliciting an individual's values, preferences and goals and is an essential HP attribute, but is not mentioned in Richardson et al.'s definition (HP knowledge, skills and competence to deliver personalised care is discussed in Chap. 3).

Box 2.1: Some Alternative Definitions of Personalised Care

1. Health care that establishes a partnership among practitioners, patients and their families (when appropriate) to ensure that decisions respect patients' wants, needs, and preferences and that patients have the education and support they need to make decisions and participate in their own care.
2. Personalised care is health care that is respectful of, and responsive to, the preferences, needs and values of patients and consumers.
3. Collaborative relationship between the person with diabetes and health professionals that results in a mutually beneficial exchange of information and shared knowledge that helps the health professional understand the individual's unique story, enables the individual to find meaning and purpose in having diabetes and develops relevant connections to achieve intentional change, transformation, personal growth and desired outcomes.
4. A person-centred health system is one that supports people to make informed decisions about, and to successfully manage, their own health and care, able to make informed decisions and choose when to invite others to act on their behalf. This required health care services to work in partnership to deliver care responsive to people's individual abilities, preferences, lifestyles and goals.

Gerteis et al. (1993a, b) described eight dimensions of personalised care:

1. Respect for the person and their preferences, values and needs.
2. Information, education and communication. This requirement refers to HPs' skills and knowledge as well as those of the individual. However people's information needs are often not met during clinical encounters (Weiner et al. 2013). The health literacy of HPs and people with diabetes influence communication.
3. Integrated, coordinated care and services, which is very challenging to achieve for older people with diabetes because of their complex care needs and 'silo' disease disciplines and guidelines.
4. Emotional support. People report that many of their emotional needs are not met (Weiner et al. 2013). Bombeke et al. (2011) found medical students' empathy and communication skills decline as they progress through their training. Haight et al. (1994) reported nurse students had more positive attitudes towards older people following 'exposure' to healthy and hospitalised older people in the first year of training. Their positivity decreased by the end of their 3 year training. Older students and those with grandparent role models had more positive attitudes to older people.

5. Physical comfort such as managing pain.
6. Involving family and friends in decisions. However, HPs should seek the consent of the individual, first.
7. Continuity among health service providers (care transition). Needs change during life transitions, which are described in Chap. 7.
8. Access to care services, which includes physical access, language, waiting time, cultural appropriateness.

Berghout et al. (2015) interviewed 34 HPs working in a geriatric department of a New York hospital to explore the individual contribution of each dimension to the whole. These HPs regarded patient preferences, information, education and coordinated care as the most important dimensions of personalised care. It is very interesting that older people were not interviewed and their views may or may not be the same as the HPs' views. It is possible they would have a different perspective and place more emphasis on the HPs' ability to communicate and deliver 'the art of care'.

Epstein and Street defined patient-centred communication as: '(1) eliciting and understanding patient perspectives: concerns, ideas, expectations, need, feelings and functioning) (2) understanding the patient and his or her unique psychosocial and cultural contexts (3) reaching a shared understanding of patient problems and treatments that are concordant with patient values'.

Epstein and Street use the word 'patient', which puts the individual in a subservient position, but their definition suggests both the HP's and the individual's agendas need to be considered through sharing information: the HP as an expert in the illness (diabetes); the individual as the expert in *their diabetes*, *their life* and the inter-related factors that are likely to affect outcomes. People with diabetes accumulate a great deal of wisdom throughout their lives and through managing their diabetes. In fact, vocabulary, knowledge and wisdom generally continue to increase in older age (Book of the Brain (author not listed) 2017).

There is a dialectical relationship between coping with adversity and developing wisdom (Linley 2003). The diagnosis of diabetes interrupts usual lifestyle and meanings the person takes for granted. If diabetes triggers the person to review their situation, adapt and change, the adversity (diabetes) can result in new knowledge, wisdom and insight into the self. That is, personal and spiritual growth can occur. Chapter 7 explores life transitions in detail.

2.3   Language and Terminology

Words are powerful. The term 'patient' suggests a power hierarchy. If HPs are to deliver personalised care and 'empower' people, they must be willing to accept their clinical knowledge, and skills might make them an expert in some respects, but not an expert in the person they are caring for and they need to be willing to relinquish some of their 'power'.

The Oxford Dictionary entry for patient states: one who tolerates delays, problems and suffering without complaint. The Cambridge Dictionary entry for patient also encompasses the notion of waiting, but uses the term person: a person receiving medical care or waiting for it. There are many negative, judgemental words in the diabetes 'dialect' such as control, good control, poor control, bad control and tight control; regime with its military connotations that reflect the control word target that people with diabetes must meet, otherwise they are non-compliant, non-adherent and end up with poor control and need tests they pass or fail depending on their blood glucose pattern and HbA1c (Diabetes Australia 2011; Dunning et al. 2017).

The doctor told me I had a weight problem. I found that so negative. I know I am overweight but I went to her for advice, her help—my weight is an opportunity for me to change. I think she has a weight problem too.

The impact of the 'diabetes dialect' on people with diabetes' feelings, reactions and outcomes is highlighted in three important publications: the Diabetes Australia Position Statement on language (2012), International Diabetes Federation Language Philosophy (2014) and Dunning et al. (2017). These language statements should inform HPs' interaction with all people with diabetes. HPs also need to be mindful of the negative impact of ageist stereotyping language and 'elder speak' when they communicate with and about older people.

The way the information is conveyed is also important. HPs use three main 'voices' (Cordell 2004):

1. Doctor voice, which is often used when conversing with and taking a health history.
2. Educator voice used when giving information.
3. Fellow Human voice, which shows empathy and is used when encouraging people to tell their story.

The three voices are complementary and are often used in the same encounter. It is important that HPs make sure their voice and verbal language are congruent with their body language. The fellow human voice might align more closely with personalised care and shared decision-making, but there is a place for all three voices. The art is to choose the 'right' voice for the situation, context and people involved in the conversation.

2.4   Personhood and Dignity

Many conflicts arise when the ideals of personalised care and their need to maintain dignity meet the realities of everyday life in care settings, even when personalised care is clearly part of an organisation's mission and values and is central to quality and safety practice standards. This is especially true in aged care facilities, which are widely regarded as residents' homes. Most people's homes do not have signs proclaiming *'cleaning in progress'* or their names on the doors. Dignity, like person-centred care, is a complex topic and is discussed in more detail in Chap. 3, which also explores metaphor in health care.

2.5 The Art of Personalising Care: What Can We Learn from Horse Whisperers and Horse Breakers?

Anybody who read *The Horse Whisperer* or saw the movie should be able to describe the difference between horse whispering and horse breaking approaches to getting horses to do what humans want. Horse whispering is a metaphor for the art of personalising care (for humans and animals). Chapter 3 discusses literary fiction and metaphors and how they apply to the art of personalising care.

2.6 The Metaphor

A horse breaker uses whips and spurs to drive horses where the breaker wants them to go. Interesting, considering a horse's first instinct when it is threatened is to run away—fast; and maybe to kick, buck, bite, if it is cornered. Are horse whips and spurs very different from HPs using scare tactics and nagging to get a person with diabetes to follow their recommendations? Scare tactics, like whips, are not very helpful and people with diabetes might not come back for follow-up appointments, or stop listening, and could end up with short- of long-term complications.

Many people know the old adage 'you can lead a horse to water but you can't make it drink'. A horse whisperer would know if you can't change the horse, you might get somewhere if you change *your* approach. For example, some readers might know the comic strip Hagar. Hagar's wife asks:

Do you know what your problems are?
I drink too much, I eat too much, I fight too much and I stay out too late.

There is no doubt that repetition is an important aspect of education: but, there is a fine line between repetition and nagging. Hagar has been nagged by his HPs, and now his wife, many times. He knows what he needs to change but:

It just saves time when I list them myself…

Hagar's HPs and his wife could change *their* nagging approach and use some nudge techniques, if they think about who Hagar is. He is a Viking. Vikings were warriors and became heroes if they fought well. If they fought well they celebrated by drinking and feasting and being rewarded with rings OR they died in battle and went to Valhalla—a key goal for Vikings.

HPs could explain to Hagar that he would have a better chance of fighting well and achieving his goal of going to Valhalla by building his muscle strength and endurance by eating well and not drinking so much alcohol, which is likely to slow his reflexes during a battle. HPs could help Hagar's wife understand that she might need to change her tactics too; given carers play a significant role in the lives of people with diabetes. That is respecting their choices and working with them.

Hagar's HPs need to build a partnership with him and his wife and to identify his values, preferences and goals and enable his wife to support his choices. Horse whisperers recognise the importance of developing a relationship with the horse so it will learn to work in partnership with them. Relationship building requires time, respect, patience and learning about one's own and the horse's capabilities, and their story. Relationship building in health care also takes time and requires shared respect and trust but it can occur in a short time if the focus is the person and not the diabetes.

A modern day Hagar

*Look!----I **know** I should eat low fat and no sugar and all that stuff and exercise. I know it's good for my diabetes.--I've heard it all before.*

Ok, let's talk about something else. Tell me what you would like to be doing in five years.

That's easy. I want to be able to play with my grandchildren, read to them, and love my wife.

What would it be like if you could not read to your grandchildren because you could not see very well?

That would be awful. I would not be much use to them or my wife then either.

How do you think you could look after your eyesight so you can do things with your family and stay well?

The man was silent for about 10 min. The HP waited quietly. The man said:

I see what you are getting at. I need to eat healthy and get of my backside so I can do things I want to do in the future. You know, nobody has ever talked about it like that before. All that diet and exercise stuff is about the diabetes but you made it about me- about me. That's different.

Was it horse whispering?

Horse whispering is an ancient art. Xenophon first described the art in *The Art of Horsemanship* in Greece 23 centuries ago (translated by Dakyn 1987). Xenophon's methods are still used: Monty Robert's, the Horse whisperer in the book of the same name, the trainers at the Spanish Riding School in Vienna and Black Caviar's trainer, Tom Moody and her Jockey Luke Nolan, all followed Xenophon's art. The riders on the cover of my copy of Xenophon's book are riding without stirrups, saddles or bridles and they are not using spurs or whips. The horses have accepted the relationship with their riders and are working in partnership *with* them—not for them!

In other words, you do not have to control or frighten a horse, or a person, to earn cooperation:

> *If you can use your skills to open a door that the horse wants to go through, then you have a horse as a willing partner instead of your unwilling subject* (Monty Roberts in Evans 1996)

All these examples show respect, common sense, listening and observing, lead to first a conversation, then an effective partnership that leads to outcomes that meet both party's needs. As indicated, these are key aspects of the art of personalising care. They require HPs to be expert communicators and reflective practitioners and listeners.

2.7   Shared Decision-Making

Shared decision-making requires the HP/HPs, the individuality diabetes and sometimes their relatives to discuss issues and come to an agreed decision. Shared decision-making is easier if there is an established trusted relationship and everybody's health literacy is considered. Shared decision-making also occurs in interdisciplinary HP teams and sometimes within families.

The promoted patient participation in care as an international priority and many countries followed suit. Shared decision-making recognises the individual's right to decisions about their life and care and is based on the key ethical principle autonomy, dignity and self-determination. It inevitably involves negotiation and compromise by all parties who need to acknowledge and accept the varied roles and expertise of the communicators.

Individuals must receive enough information in a format suitable to their learning style, literacy and numeracy, cognitive capacity and the topic under discussion to be able to actively participate and make informed decisions. People who are actively involved in decisions are more likely to 'own' their decisions, adhere to treatment and have better outcomes.

There are also psychological, ethical and legal reason for providing information about potential benefits, risks, complications and side effects of different courses of treatment for their particular illness, including fewer complaints about care and care providers. Well-informed people can prepare themselves for future events and reduce uncertainty by identifying adverse events early and taking appropriate action to reduce the risks (Case et al. 2005).

People have the ultimate choice about what happens to their bodies: they can only make informed choices if they have all the relevant information in a format they can understand. HPs need to accept that not everybody wants to or is able to make care decisions. Thus, it is important to determine the role people want to play in their care, rather than assuming everybody will participate in decision-making on the basis of the current mantra about 'engaged consumers' or more recent jargon 'activated patients/consumers'.

We can even measure patient activation using the Patient Activation Measure (PAM) (Hibbard 2008). Knowing a person's PAM score can be very helpful, if it is used in context and takes account of the individual's health and other factors at the time. It is not helpful to label a person according to some level and trying to change people who do not meet the required level. It is more important to understand their reasons for participating or not participating.

Flynn et al. (2006) used a questionnaire from the Wisconsin Longitudinal Study with some additional questions to determine preferences for four components of the decision-making process relating to physician's: knowledge about the patients history, disclosure of treatment choices, discussing treatment choice, and selecting a treatment ($n = 5199$).

Fifty-seven percent wanted control over all important medical decisions 'autonomists', 81% preferred to discuss treatment with their doctors; 39% wanted their physician to make important medical decisions 'delegators', and 41% preferred to discuss treatment choices. Most wanted their physicians to know everything about their medical history and to be given choices. People with higher education, women and those taking fewer prescription medicines were more likely to want to be actively involved in decision-making.

Similarly, Chewning et al. (2012) reviewed papers published between 1980 and 2007 that examined the role people wanted to play in their care. They identified three groups:

1. People who wanted to delegate decisions to their doctors.
2. Those who wanted to share decision-making.
3. Those who wanted to make decisions themselves (alone).

However, labelling people is unhelpful and misleading. Individuals have different desires for the different components of the decision-making process and differing capacity to participate at different times Willingness to participate depends on a number of demographic variables including age, gender, health status and education (Say et al. 2006).

2.8   Health Literacy

Health literacy refers to basic reading and numerical skills that enable individuals to function in their health and social environments (Safeer and Keenan 2003). It is a multifaceted concept that encompasses obtaining, understanding and processing basic health information required to make appropriate informed decisions. Health literacy depends on many factors including education, culture, health status, complexity and design of information.

Most individual read at eighth grade level, but 20% of most participants read below 5th grade level. Significantly, most health information is written at least grade 10. Many people older than age 60 have inadequate health literacy (Ridpath et al. 2007). Readability is further compromised by colours contrast, layout, the amount of white space around text, the size of the chunks of text (paragraphs) and font size and type.

Low reading skills and suboptimal health outcomes are related. These issues are compounded for people whose first language is not English. I acknowledge the language bias in that comment. The same issues apply in all cultures.

HPs often believe people's health literacy level is higher than it actually is, especially if the person is a professional and/or a colleague. Likewise, people become adept at hiding their literacy problems. Behaviours that suggest an individual has inadequate health literacy skills are:

• Asking for help to complete forms.
• Being accompanied to appointments by a literate family member, friend or interpreter.
• Inability to keep appointments.
• Making excuses such as I forgot my glasses/hearing aids, although it is important to check that people who need these aids have them before beginning any health appointment or education.
• Inadequate adherence to recommendations.

- Postponing decisions 'I will read it when I get home'.

Various types of health literacy are described (Stacey et al. 2016):

Functional: basic reading and writing skills and ability to understand information. It includes numerical literacy, e.g. ability to correctly dial up an insulin dose on an insulin pen device.

Interactive: ability to communicate with others and extract information and discuss it and to share personal values, goals, preferences and health concerns.

Critical: requires advanced cognitive skills such as the capacity to analyse information and make decisions using the information. Hypo- and hyperglycaemia affect cognition and an older person may have cognitive changes that affect critical health literacy periodically or permanently (Chaps. 1 and 8). Cognitive changes do not mean the individual cannot engage in conversations. The art is to present information in a way that suits the individual and that can change from time to time.

A number of strategies can be used to enhance shared decision-making, including using guidelines and decision-aids (Chap. 4), discussion to clarify the individual's values and preferences, coaching older people with diabetes and HPs I the art of making decisions, asking good question a prompt sheet. These may be written, electronic or audio but they must conform to standards for language, design and layout.

2.9   Information, Knowledge and Memory

Information is a meaningful, sharable common pattern (MacFarlane 2013). Humans evolved as a species and learned collectively and individually to recognise and ascribe meaning to patterns, including linguistic patterns. Information consists of a triad of components: mental, social and physical. The social aspects of information are very important to education and health consultations where information is shared. Some knowledge is innate, but most is gained through interacting with the world and other people. Each interaction generates new information that is encoded and stored as memory and can be retrieved when relevant.

Only explicit language-based knowledge can be transmitted in written form and via technology (explicit knowledge). A great deal of knowledge is tacit knowledge and not expressed in language: 'we know but we cannot tell it'. Likewise, people's tacit knowledge is difficult to assess. Brainstorming and group education programmes enable stored and tacit knowledge to surface, shared and discussed. Modern day Hagar's story has elements of sharing tacit knowledge and brainstorming to reach understanding.

Learning and using information involves several inter-related sensory and cognitive processes, including the ability to:

- Hear and see information.
- Understand the information.
- Absorb new information.

- Make connections between stored information and new information synthesise it and make comparisons to create new knowledge.
- Remember the information and be able to retrieve (recall) it when needed.
- Use the information (Stevens and Osborne 2003).

Many factors individually and collectively affect those processes, including ageing. Ageing affects the speed of mental processing, cognitive flexibility, capacity to make inferences from the information and to manage several types of information simultaneously (multitask) and to focus. Older people have less working memory, the mind's capacity at any given moment, than younger people. Consequently, older people are more likely to become cognitively fatigues during long education and consultation sessions and cognitive assessment process such as trying to understand complex information.

Knowledge is retained across the lifespan although cognitive capacity can be affected by age and disease states. Thus, older people often have extensive knowledge base and considerable experience and insight to bring shared decision-making. They make decisions differently from young people but the actual decisions are often similar (Yates and Patalano 1999). Older people review less information, eliminate choices faster and are less likely to analyse information while making decisions. They also often make decision using 'rules' such as 'do not take medicines that cause side effect' and rely on past experiences to inform their decisions.

The way information is organised and presented influences whether older people are willing and able to read and use it.

Now the annoying thing about scholars [HPs] *is that they always use BIG WORDS... and sometimes one gets the impression those BIG WORDS are there to keep us from understanding* (The Tao of Pooh and the Te of Piglet Hoff 2008).

General strategies for preparing information are to:

- Know the audience/s and tailor the information to the audience, and more importantly, ensure it can be tailored for individuals.
- Understand the individual's motivation and readiness to learn.
- Limit the amount and complexity of information in key messages and choices.
- Use concrete information and examples.
- Define terms or use 'plain language'.
- Draw on the person's experiences. That can only be achieved by carefully listening to the person's story.
- Use stories, poems and pictures.
- Ensure the environment is conducive to learning (Stevens & Osbourne 2003).

2.10   Personalised Care

... the highly scientific development of this mechanistic age had led perhaps to some loss in appreciation of the individuality of the patient and trusting largely to laboratories and outside agencies which tended to make the patient, not the hub of the wheel but the spoke

We can ask whether some research that relies on randomisation and control might actually regress people to the mean. The answer might be yes, especially for older people—depending on the way HPs use the research and resultant guidelines and algorithms that often become reduced to 'tick boxes' that signify present/absent or done/not done (Chaps. 4 and 10). Most recent 'diabetes' guidelines and education strategies recommend individualising targets to suit the person, but the targets largely refer to metabolic parameters such as HbA1c and people with diabetes often find the word 'target' challenging (DA 2011; Dunning et al. 2017). Significantly, most do not actually tell HPs how to apply the guidelines or research evidence in practice.

Martin mentioned placing the patient at the hub of the wheel, nowadays we use the term placing the person at the centre of care so-called person-centred care, which often sounds like personscented care, it rolls of the tongue so glibly. We use diagrams showing services and HPs revolving around the individual like a halo. Is that truly person-centred OR is it an entrapment model?

If you ask a person with diabetes what person-centred care looks like, especially if you ask them to draw it, they describe a more encompassing model that includes things important to them besides health care organisations and HPs. It includes their connections with other people and their environment, their pets and gardens. Developing an Ecomap and/or a Genomap with the individual as part of an holistic assessment is a more person-centred approach and can contribute vital information *about the person* that can inform their care plan (Table 2.1).

When preparing my lecture in 2016 and revisiting the literature review for this book I asked 20 randomly encountered older people with diabetes 'What things are important to you when you see a health professional'. Important things were:

- To be treated as a unique individual with a life story and for the HP to understand diabetes in only one part of who I am.
- Trust and to feel comfortable and be treated like an equal.
- HPs to be 'real people' who listen and do not impose their views on me and other people.
- HPs who are honest and respectful.
- To meet HPs in a 'nice environment' that is quiet and not cluttered where I do not feel rushed or like I am competing with a computer.
- HPs plan for my visit and have all my information ready—they are ready for ME.

2.11   Measuring Personalised Care

A range of processes can be used but they must be fit for purpose and relate to the purpose of the evaluation. An evaluation should include process evaluation as well as other measures and might include PROMs. Evaluation strategies generally include patient satisfaction and patient experience using questionnaires, HP surveys collected via interviews, self-completed forms and observation. Data can be collected from Risk man and complaints as well as medical record audits.

Table 2.1 Some 'criteria' people with diabetes, health professionals and organisations need to facilitate personalised diabetes care

Person with diabetes	Health professional	Organisations
Relevant health literacy and numeracy	Relevant health literacy and numeracy	Embed personalised care (PC) in organisation mission and values and strategic plan
Access to relevant information in a format that meets their needs and at a time that suits their needs	Emotional intelligence	
	Reflective practitioners	Clearly communicate these throughout the organisation, other service providers and to consumers
	Relevant knowledge and skills, which they keep current thorough continued learning and reflection	
The knowledge and capabilities to seek information and apply it to their diabetes care		Include PC in HP position descriptions
	Exemplary communicators (horse whisperers) able to actively listen, ask relevant questions	Employ leaders who demonstrate PC (appropriate role models)
Become experts in their diabetes		Develop an environment that supports PC with relevant referral pathways and collaborative relationships
	Understand when people are not able or do not want to participate in shared decision-making and act in the best interests of the individual at those times	
Accept they have responsibilities as well as rights		Technology to support PC
Accept the consequences of their choices		Processes to measure outcomes, impact and collect feedback from all users and providers
	Accept the person's choices, even when they are not the choice the HP recommends	
	Identify the individual's issues and their values, goals and preferences	
	Monitor outcomes relevant to the individual	
	Develop and maintain a therapeutic relationship	

Over 50 tools are used to measure the various concepts that underpin personalised care including:

- Individual care scale
- Measure of Process of Care
- Person-centred Assessment Tool
- Self-Assessment Tool—Clinical Practice
- The Dimensional Wisdom Model (Ardelt 2011) can be used to measure personal wisdom. It includes cognitive, reflective and benevolent dimensions and addresses most explicit (expert) and implicit or lay wisdom.

However, a significant challenge is having a usable way to measure HPs' ability to listen and respond to people with diabetes and the public. More than one measurement process might be needed depending on the aim of the evaluation.

We also need to consider the implications of the Human Genome Project for personalised medicine and care and how the ability to predict disease development and target therapies will influence personalised care and the skills HPs need to encompass these rapidly approaching changes. Two areas of study will be particularly pertinent to older people: diabetes and dementia. These issues are discussed in more detail in Chap. 6.

2.12 Summary

In summary, and to return to the horse whisperer, people with diabetes are more likely to engage with HPs and make appropriate choice/decisions if their HPs are excellent communicators, especially in the art of *didirri* listening exemplified by Monty Roberts:

> *I sought a non-violent way of communicating my intent while respecting the horse's rights. It was up to me to listen, to read the signals, and show that I understood the horse's language by the accuracy of my response* (Roberts 1996)

I leave the final words to Luke Nolan, Black Caviar's jockey. There was a very strong relationship between Nolan and Black Caviar. He knew her very well and she trusted him. Her 22nd consecutive win in the diamond Jubilee Stakes at Royal Ascot was the stuff of legends. Nolan knew Black Caviar was still suffering from jet lag when she raced that day, she lost weight during the trip and had not acclimatised to the UK. Her coat was not in good condition and she had ligament injuries that caused pain when she extended into a gallop.

Black caviar only just won that day. If you watch a replay of the race you can see when Nolan stopped riding and Black Caviar slows down. Nolan said:

> *I knew she was nowhere near her best. She had done enough. I could see the finish line. I knew I would annoy her if I kept riding her to the line. She is special, a special horse to me. I've never wanted to annoy her.*

> *I held my hands at the base of her neck and she knew we were done.*

They were out in front, the winning post was in sight and Nolan gave her permission to slow down (resting his hands at the base of her neck). Then he realised there was a horse on his shoulder coming up fast. He said:

> *I gave her neck a rub, I knew she was completely spent, but she flattened and stretched out her glorious neck and that was all that was required. She did that for me* (Whateley 2012)

2.13   Reflection Points

1. Reflect on your understanding of personalised care. Has it changed in any way since reading this chapter?
2. Think about the common elements in the definitions in Box 2.1: how are they similar and how are they different?
3. What did you learn about communication and partnerships from Luke Nolan and Black Caviar?

References

Ardelt M (2011) Wisdom, age and well-being. In: Scaie K, Willis S (eds) Handbook of psychology of ageing. Elsevier, Amsterdam, pp 279–291

Bensing J (2000) Bridging the gap. Separate worlds of evidence-based medicine and patient-centred medicine. Patient Educ Couns 39:17–25. https://doi.org/10.1016/S0738-3991(99)00087-7

Berghout M, Van Exel J, Leensvaart L et al (2015) Healthcare professionals' views on patient-centered care in hospitals. BMC Health Serv Res 15:385. https://doi.org/10.1186/s12913-015-1049-z

Bombeke V, Van Roosbroeck S, De Winter B et al (2011) Medical students trained in communication skills show a decline in patient-centred attitudes: an observational study comparing two cohorts during clinical clerkships. Patient Educ Couns 84(3):310–318. https://doi.org/10.1016/j.pec.2011.03.007

Case D, Andrews J, Johnson J, Allard S (2005) Avoiding versus seeking: the relationship of information seeking to avoidance, blunting, coping, dissonance, and related concepts. J Med Libr Assoc 93:353–362

Chewning B, Bylund C, Shah B, Arora N, Gueguen J, Makoul G (2012) Patient preferences for shared decisions: a systematic review. Patient Educ Couns 86:9–18. https://doi.org/10.1016/j.pec.2011.02.004

Cordell M (2004) The Dynamic Consultation: A discourse analytical study of doctor ... https://books.google.com/books/about/The_Dynamic_Consultation.html?id, https://doi.org/10.1136/jramc-150-04-04

Coulter A, Entwhistle V, Eccles A et al (2015) Personalised care planning for adults with chronic long term health conditions. Cochrane Syst Rev. https://doi.org/10.1002/1465185.c001523.pub2

Diabetes Australia (DA) (2011) A new language for diabetes: improving communication with and about people with diabetes. DA, Canberra

Dunning T, Speight J, Bennett C (2017) Language, the 'diabetes restricted code/dialect,' and what it means for people with diabetes and clinicians. Diabetes Educ 47(1):18–26

Flynn K, Smith M, Vanness D (2006) A typology of preferences for participation in health care decision making. Soc Sci Med 53(5):1156–1169

Frederikson L (1995) Exploring information-exchange in consultations: patients' view of performance and outcomes. Patient Educ Couns 25:237–246. https://doi.org/10.1016/0738-3991(95)00801-6

Gerteis M, Edgman-Levitan S, Walker J et al (1993a) What patients really want. Health Manage Q 15(3):2–6

Gerteis M, Edgman-Levitan S, Daly J, Delbanco T (1993b) Through the patient's eyes: understanding and promoting patient-centered care. Jossey-Bass, San Francisco

Glas R (1996) The patient-physician relationship. J Am Med Assoc 275:147–148

Hagar The Horrible—Unhealthy Comics And Cartoons… (n.d.) www.cartoonistgroup.com/…/The-Unhealthy-Comics-and-Cartoons-by-Hagar+The+Horrible.php

Haight BK, Christ MA, Dias JK (1994) Does nursing education promote ageism? J Adv Nurs 20:382–390. https://doi.org/10.1046/j.1365-2648.1994.20020382.x

Hibbard J (2008) Can increasing patient activation improve the outcomes of care? Presentation university of Oregon. https://doi.org/10.1603/0046-225X-37.6.1558

Hoff B (2008) The Tao of Pooh and the Te of Piglet. Egemont Publishing UK Ltd, London. https://doi.org/10.1371/journal.pbio.0060313

International Diabetes Federation (IDF) (2014) Language Philosophy. www.idf.org

Karr M (undated, 1994) The moment of death. In: Downie R (ed) The healing arts: an Oxford illustrated anthology. Oxford University Press, Oxford, pp 191–198

Linley P (2003) Positive adaptation to trauma wisdom as both process and outcome. Journal Trauma Stress 16(6):601–610. https://doi.org/10.1023/B:JOTS.0000004086.64509.09

MacFarlane A (2013) Information, knowledge and intelligence. Philosophy Now, October 18–20

Rathert C, Wyrwich M, Boren S (2013) Patient-centered care and outcomes: a systematic review of the literature. Med Care Res Rev 70(4):351–379

Richardson W, Berwick D, Bisgard J, Institute of Medicine et al (2001) Crossing the quality chasm: a new system for the 21st century. National Academy Press, Washington. https://doi.org/10.1086/319196

Ridpath J, Green R, Wiese C (2007) PRISM readability toolkit, 3rd edition. Seattle. J Am Med Assoc 305:1130–1131

Roberts M (1996) The Horse Whisperer. Dell Publishing, New York

Safeer R, Keenan I (2003) Health literacy: the gap between physicians and patients. Am Fam Physician 72(3):463–468

Say R, Murtagh M, Thomson R (2006) Patients' preference for involvement in medical decision making: a narrative review. Patient Educ Couns 60(2):102–114. https://doi.org/10.1016/j.pec.2005.02.003

Starfield B (2011) Is patient-centred care the same as person-focused care. Permanente J 15(2):63–69

Stevens B, Osborne H (2003) Communicating with clients in person and over the phone. Issue Brief Cent Medicare Educ 4(8):1–8

Weiner S, Schwatz A, Sharma G et al (2013) Patient-centered decision making and health care outcomes: an observational study. Ann Intern Med 158(8):573–579. https://doi.org/10.7326/0003-4819-158-8-201304160-00001

Whateley G (2012) Black Caviar. Harper Collins. Sydney

Xenophon (1987) On Horsemanship translated by Dakyn H. MacMillan. https://doi.org/10.17226/991

Yates J, Patalano A (1999) Decision-making and ageing patients; Cognition and human factors perspectives. Lawrence Erlbaum, Mahwa, pp 31–54. https://doi.org/10.1080/01971529909349312

Health Professionals: What Do They Need to Cogenerate Holistic Personalised Care?

3

Trisha Dunning and Mark Kennedy

> *Perdu collected the words that stood out from the stream of everyday expressions. The shining words were the ones that revealed how this woman saw and smelled and felt. What was really important to her, what bothered her, and how she was feeling right now? What she wished to conceal behind a fog of words. Pains and longings.*
>
> *Monsieur Perdu fished out these words....Yet that was only part of what Perdu listened out for and recorded: what made the soul unhappy. Then, there was the second part: what makes the soul happy. Monsieur Perdu knew that the texture of the things the person loves rubs off in his or her language.*
>
> *(George 2015)*

Key Points

- The ability to '*Listen Like a Dog*' (Lazarus 2016) is essential to holistic personalised care.
- Health professionals must reflect in and on their values, attitudes and beliefs as well as their practice to enhance their skills and insight.
- Self-knowledge, creativity and open mindedness are as important as academic and technical skills and knowledge—possibly more important.
- Inclusive collaboration is essential.

T. Dunning, A.M., M.Ed., Ph.D., R.N., C.D.E.
Centre for Quality and Patient Safety Research, Barwon Health Partnership, Deakin University, Geelong, VIC, Australia
e-mail: trisha.dunning@barwonhealth.org.au; trisha.dunning@deakin.edu.au

M. Kennedy (✉)
Department of General Practice, University of Melbourne, Geelong, VIC, Australia

3.1   Introduction

Many papers and guidelines describe core diabetes management interventions and strategies and often refer to education goals such as empowering people with diabetes, educating them, and supporting them to make behaviour changes to undertake self-care: a life time of self-care that can become increasingly burdensome as people grow older. The self-care burden adds to associated burdens: living with diabetes (physical, psychological and social) and medicine-related burden. A big assumption in that list is that the person actually needs to change their behaviour. That might not be the case: the Health professional (HP) maybe the one who needs to change to help older people and their families (see Chap. 2). The art of listening like a dog could help HPs understand whether they need to change their strategies/approach and make their mark on the world, or at least on the person they are interacting with.

Significantly, clinical guidelines do not usually indicate what values, attitudes, beliefs, knowledge and competence HPs need or the type of role model they need to present—and that is not their purpose. We can make some inferences about required knowledge and competence from guidelines and research. Some of competencies, attitudes and skills are included in regulatory and professional frameworks and codes, 'competency documents', discipline registration requirements and continuing professional development portfolios. Others are not included because they are not considered and/or because they are hard to define and measure. These hard-to-define aspects are explored in this chapter.

3.2   Credentialing, Frameworks and Models

HP credentialing has become important to many service providers to enable them to demonstrate their workforce is appropriately prepared to provide quality care. Initial qualifications are the beginning of lifelong learning (Hickey et al. 2013). Credentialed status implies extra training and expertise in some specific aspects of care such as diabetes education.

The term 'credentialing' means different things in different countries. Some countries such as Australia apply credentialing to people and use the terms 'accreditation' or 'recognition' for programmes and organisations. Other countries use credentialing to refer to the requirements and evaluation processes individuals and organisations must meet for various reasons including practising and continuing to offer services. Some of these credentialing requirements include personalised care.

Many diabetes care models, clinical guidelines and position statements throughout the world encompass elements of personalised care, for example, The Empowerment Model, Chronic Disease Models, Peer Education, Conversation Maps and the American Association of Diabetes Educators (AADE) Diabetes Self-Management Model. These may or may not be suitable for older people. Some are idealistic, even when they are practical and likely to benefit older people with diabetes. Most do not have robust measures of HPs' competence to deliver personalised care, other than knowledge and/or HbA1c, which are actually surrogate markers of HP performance, and indeed of older people with diabetes 'performance'. Increasingly, the literature suggests HbA1c might no longer be the 'Gold Standard' outcome measure of 'everything'.

Knowledge-practice gaps are well described in the literature and are outlined in Chaps. 4 and 10. Various reasons have been postulated for the gap, and have not changed in over 20 years (Yassin 1994). Some HP-related barriers include HPs not:

- Knowing the guidance exists
- Having ready access to guidance in written and electronic formats
- Knowing how to apply the recommendations to the individuals they care for.

Some strategies HPs could use to implement guideline recommendations are discussed in Chap. 4. Personalised care could be the balance point between idealistic care (evidence) and realistic care (what is possible for each individual in each specific situation). Creativity and lateral thinking, including outside 'health', could help HPs find innovative ways to personalise care, like the architect, Seidler, who 'choose the path less travelled':

> *Architecture isn't about style. It's about contemporary means and methods and how we can articulate that with clarity. We will never progress if we always try to imitate our neighbour* (Harry Seidler in Lacey 2013)

Seidler's choice to do dare to be different from the architectural style of the time required commitment and courage. It made all the difference for him. However, it is important to choose carefully, after all, well-trodden paths have shown the way for centuries and led to new discoveries and change. We are suggesting health professionals (HP) have the courage to try something different and hope they find some ideas and inspiration in this book to help them do so.

Appreciative Inquiry might be a new look at a well-trodden path for HPS. It emerged in the 1980s to improve organisational performance (Acosta and Douthwaite 2005). Key elements of the model can be applied to personalising health care. Appreciative Inquiry is a way of thinking and working to foster reflection on what organisations need to do, or in this case what HPs need to know and do to help older people with diabetes communicate their needs. Appreciative Inquiry contains many HPs use to document a medical history that can be applied to personalising diabetes care such as:

- Establishing the focus of the inquiry by using open but relevant first question, e.g. 'Tell me a story about a time when you were able to'.
- Using probing and clarifying questions to elicit important aspects of the story as well as undertaking relevant assessments at a pertinent time that does not affect/interrupt the story. Interruptions could cause the person to leave out important elements of the story that influence the care and education they need.
- Listening to the language and words the person uses: words and the way individuals use words are part of the story and can help HPs choose words the person is likely to understand and/or engage with.

- Summarising the story and using the person's accumulated wisdom contained within the story to co-design care with the individual (shared decision-making).
- Making it happen together by developing an implementation plan.

The authors acknowledge, but do not focus on, the 'standard' diabetes knowledge and competence described in HP education curricula and professional organisation documents such as the American Association of Diabetes Educators, The Australian Diabetes Educators Association and similar documents of other health disciplines. Likewise, it does not specifically describe the roles of various HP disciplines or their scopes of practice. Roles and scopes of practice are not fixed for all time, they continually evolve. The authors acknowledge there are different expectations of beginning and experienced practitioners.

The aim of the chapter is to challenge HPs to reflect outside their knowledge and competency 'squares' or comfort zones, to be creative and flexible in their approach to each individual with diabetes and to reflect on how they can provide conditions in which personalised care and education plans can be co-created with older people with diabetes.

3.3 Inspirational Albert Einstein

Albert Einstein stated:

I never teach my pupils: I only attempt to provide the conditions in which they can learn.

The statement illustrates the fact that HPs are not in control of what people learn, or how they value, interpret and use the information they acquire. It does not imply the HP/teacher gives people knowledge. It promotes learning as an active process. One can share knowledge with another person by giving them information—the person creates their own knowledge from the information they acquire via complex processes in the brain.

Einstein also suggested one person cannot empower another, but providing conditions in which people feel safe to learn and to disclose information can help the person empower themselves. The notion that one could empower another person reflects doing things to people rather than with them, as the term 'shared decision-making' implies. That is not to say empowerment is not important. It is. The way words are used and how the principles of shared decision-making and personalised care are applied in education and care are essential aspects of effective communication. HPs must use language that matches their intent and actions (see Chap. 2).

The quote also suggests that the conditions in which teaching and care planning are delivered are important, and affect outcomes. The situation might require other people such as family carers and interpreters to be involved, which changes the dynamics of the situation and the relationships within it. It highlights the fact that the teacher, in this case the HP, needs to actively find out what conditions suit the individual *at that specific time* and their learning style in order to create conditions that help them learn.

Computer-generated 'personalised' care plans are becoming an increasingly common part of 'the situation'. Sadly these are often not, in fact, truly personalised:

The woman was angry. She threw some papers at me and shouted:

I don't know what this means. The doctor gave it to me after five minutes and said there is your diabetes goals and plan—do you have any questions. I got the feeling I should not waste his time so I left. He just gave it to me. He did not bother to ask what I wanted. Can you tell me what it means?

'It' was an electronic care plan created by her GP or practice nurse and given to her by her GP during a routine diabetes monitoring consultation. According to the plan, one of **her** care goals was to reduce her alcohol intake to one glass per day.

What!!!!. Once glass a day is it????

I'm an alcoholic! I've not had alcohol for five years. Now I have to have one glass every day!!! That plan is useless and has nothing to do with me.

What a difference a taking a comprehensive history, asking appropriate questions and using sensitive probing and clarifying questions could have made. But, we do not actually know whether the GP or practice nurse did use these skills? We only have a small piece of the total situation, the woman's story—not enough to make judgements about the encounter.

One can make some assumptions about what attitudes, knowledge and skills HPs need to engage with people in order to personalise care with them from the preceding discussion. Note the deliberate use of the word 'with', in preference to 'for' in the woman's last statement and in the title of the book. 'With' reflects personalised care; 'for' does not. Likewise, 'for' is disempowering language.

All that from a short quote?! It is an example of reflection on practice. HPs also need to be able to reflect in practice.

3.4   What Do Health Professionals Need to Create Conditions in Which Older People with Diabetes Can Actively Engage in Their Care?

The words 'knowledge', 'competence' and 'skills' are deliberately missing from the question because these terms do not overtly encompass, attitudes, behaviours and beliefs, which are as important, maybe more important, than knowledge and competence. Knowledge, skills and competence can be learned and change over time as HPs gain experience and practice changes through research and technology. It is much harder to change attitudes and beliefs, as most HPs realise; yet HPs' attitudes and beliefs have a big impact on older people with diabetes' outcomes (Nam et al. 2011).

Helping the individual be an active partner in the care process requires supportive HP language, coaching, negotiating, maybe even nudging, rather than directive behaviours. Many HPs regard engaging with people to co-create care plans too time consuming or not suitable for or important to all individuals (Nam et al. 2011). Often the opportunity to work with an individual to develop an appropriate care plan based on the individual's attitudes, beliefs, priorities and needs at a particular point in time is lost because the immediate reason for the consultation is procedural rather than on establishing shared management and care goals. It must also be acknowledged that not all older people want to engage in shared decision-making and some are not able to participate (Chaps. 2 and 4).

Interestingly, using a narrative approach does not actually take a lot of time. Langewitz et al. (2002) undertook a study involving 335 people with complex medical histories in general practice and showed 2 min of active listening in consultations was long enough to identify 80% of people's concerns. Only seven of the 335 needed more than 5 min. Admittedly, the general practitioners in Langewitz et al.'s study were trained in active listening. Maybe to Listen Like a Dog (Lazarus 2016).

Education policies and curricula define qualified and professional practice and competence HPs and other professionals require as well as the need to engage in continuing professional development. However, focusing on technical skills and mastering a body of knowledge is not sufficient (Arias-Carballal 2017). Arias-Carballal (2017) was referring to school teachers' personal-emotional identity and its relationship to their professional identity. Her discourse also applies to HPs.

Diabetes education and management, like teaching, is an emotional and social endeavour, especially where personalising care is involved. Diabetes care is connected to the HP's personal life, their experience and their relationships, including relationships with people with diabetes and colleagues and shapes their knowledge, skills and behaviours. Emotional and professional identity can be enhanced by reflection in and on practice.

Thus, the HP must consider his or her personal characteristics when deciding what competencies and attitudes he or she needs to develop to deliver personalised care; for example, enthusiasm, sense of humour, ability to listen, flexibility, honesty, sensitivity, creativity and humility. Some of these characteristics are innate, most can be developed as the HP grows in experience and wisdom and reflects in and on his or her practice.

> Inspector Sullivan: *Perhaps you should think about leaving things to the professionals from now on.*
> Father Brown: *Never forget that professionals built the Titanic but an amateur built the Ark.*
> (Father Brown 2014)

HPs who have diabetes also end to consider how their experience with diabetes could affect how they relate to older people with diabetes. Such reflections are akin to the reflexive process qualitative researchers undertake and is a key aspect of the credibility of the study. Some issues to consider are:

- Whether and when to disclose their diabetes.
- The positive and negative effects of disclosure on the relationship.
- The language they use, e.g. *I know how you feel* might not be appropriate; we can never truly know what another person feels.
- Whether HPs with diabetes act as 'peer educators' when caring for people with diabetes and the personal and professional aspects of such relationships.

3.5   Reflective Practice

Reflection is essential to professional competence and the capacity to integrate theory into practice (Mann et al. 2009). Reflection is essential to *praxis*, which means action with reflection and learning by doing. *Praxis* is doing with inbuilt reflection. Most people reflect automatically, but purposeful reflection helps HPs reflect in as well as on action; the latter is a more advanced skill to develop.

Reflection helps HPS identify their personal beliefs, attitudes and values, how they developed and how they affect their practice. Learning through reflection involves HPs processing an experience several ways to explore and understand their actions, the experience and the impact it had on themselves and others. It is one way of recognising patterns, and avoid making the same mistake again, consolidates learning and the ability to use effective strategies in similar situations.

HPs could reflect on the ways they interact with older people with diabetes and families; for example, the way they:

- Could help older people and families use reflection to improve their understanding of diabetes
- Show they are actively listening
- Ask and respond to questions
- Interpret and use people's stories
- Create situations in which people feel safe to share information
- Work collaboratively with colleagues
- Identify their learning needs
- Show they are willing to question their practice
- Consider the impact of their attitudes on their behaviour and interactions with other people.

The following conversation demonstrates how one communicator negotiated an 'ocean of unspoken' and spoken messages to achieve a successful outcome and a mutually agreed solution with a reluctant learner:

> *Me explain it:* said Pooh *behind his paw.*
> *Well yes—I thought that might be nice.*
> *Well I thought it would be better if you did somehow.*
> *I don't think that is such a good idea. Said Pooh.*
> *Why not?*
> *Because when I explain things, they get in wrong places, he said, That's why.*
> *All right, I'll explain it. But you can help out every now and again. How does that sound?*
> *That's much more like it* said Pooh.
> (Hoff 1982)

HPs' attitudes and beliefs and skills affect the way they care for older people with diabetes and help them maintain or enhance their dignity and autonomy (Lothian and Philp 2001). Key attitudes and beliefs are:

Attitudes
- Respect for persons and their autonomy and dignity.
- Capacity to put aside ageist attitudes and language. Research show many HPs have pessimistic views about older people and use stereotypical and ageist language
- Willingness to consider learning from and areas outside health care such as writing, music, theatre and art. Jean-Phillip and Tizanai Assal in Switzerland led the way in incorporating the arts into diabetes education (Assal and Assal 2013).
- Commitment to ethical, professional practice.

Beliefs
- Belief in self and the need for personal self-care.
- Belief in the value of personalised care and engaging with people to co-develop care plans, when possible.
- In the value of continued professional development and self-reflection to improve practice.

Skills can be general or domain specific. General skills include organisation, leadership and management. Some domain-specific skills are discussed in the next section.

3.6 Skills and Behaviours

Skills can be general or domain specific. General skills include organisation, leadership and management. Dome domain-specific skills are discussed in this section. Of these, communication is the greatest.

'An ocean of unspoken messages' separates health professional and people with diabetes' worlds (Barabino et al. 2009). Communication is a core skill HPs need to enable them to engage in person-centred care, especially being truly present with the person and listening in silence (*Didirri*). *Didirri* is an Australian Aboriginal Term meaning inner, deep listening and quiet, still awareness and waiting. It means 'tuning in' and experiencing with the specific aim of coming to a deeper understanding of nature. It encompasses spirituality, a key, yet neglected, aspect of diabetes care.

Didirri is the type of listening HPs need to practice and become competent in. *Didirri* can be enhanced through regular meditation. HPs are often time poor and can struggle to listen intently without interrupting the person's flow of words to ask specific questions about a particular point. These frequent interruptions often prevent the person from providing important information about concerns, additional issues and barriers to self-care and compromises the development of a relevant and meaningful care plan.

Evidence suggests there are positive associations between physician communication behaviours and 'patient' outcomes, particularly recall, understanding and adherence to therapy (King and Hoppe 2013). Yet people report that physicians do not meet a significant proportion of their information needs (Weiner et al. 2013).

Some experts attribute this finding to the limited HP training in interpersonal skills. Such training occurs early in the medical curriculum but is often not reinforced in the later stages of training (Bombeke et al. 2011). Similar findings are reported in other HP disciplines; for example, Haight et al. (1994) found a gradual decline in student nurses' attitudes to older people over the 3 year training programme.

Choudhry and Fletcher (2006) reviewed 62 publications that included time in practice and age as factors that could influence practice. They found factual knowledge and adherence to appropriate standards of care tended to decline with experience; 52% of publications reported worse performance with increasing experience and 21% reported decreasing performance in some aspects of practice with no counterbalancing improvements. It is possible similar tends occur in other disciplines. The findings suggest that older HPs might need to actively reflect on these aspects of their practice and/or seek feedback from trusted colleagues and the people they care for (performance appraisal/professional development activities).

Communication is most effective if it is simple, specific, uses repetition, limits use of jargon, meets the individual's needs at the time, and the HP checks for understanding. Effective communication is a composite of several skills:

- Developing and fostering a relationship.
- Collecting information.
- Providing information
- Making decisions (hopefully with the individual if possible)
- Responding to emotions
- Knowing when and how to use probing and clarifying questions and to reflect back.
- Enabling disease and treatment behaviours.

Technology has changed the way people communicate and new ways of working besides face-to-face are emerging. There are advantages and disadvantages of using technology and these are discussed in Chap. 9.

Other important skills and behaviours HPs need beside communication include:

- The ability to create therapeutic relationships, which largely depends on the following skills.
- The capacity to look at themselves and others from a broad perspective, which encompasses reflection and reflexivity.
- The ability to 'pay attention to your intentions' (Deepak Chopra). Attention is a learned skill and refers to focused awareness. It encompasses being centred and focusing on what the person wants/desires/goals.
- The ability to listen, hear and interpret peoples' stories and use the information to plan care with them. Reading literacy fiction builds Theory of Mind (pp xx) and helps health professionals understand other peoples' mental states, which is needed to develop therapeutic relationships (Kidd and Castano 2013).
- Knowledge of teaching and learning theories, how to apply them, and how to create safe learning environments: that is, create the conditions in which students can learn.
- The ability to manage without technology—but to use technology effectively when it is relevant (Chap. 9).

3.7 Knowledge

Focusing on technical skills and diabetes knowledge and competencies is not sufficient to achieve personalised care and outcomes. Knowledge is enhanced by continual learning, repetition, reflection and using the knowledge. In addition, HPs need:

- Knowledge of self.
- Exemplary listening and other communication skills.
- Cultural competence: knowledge about cultural norms and how to work with interpreters when indicated (see page xx).
- To understanding of diabetes pathophysiology, management and complications, relationship between memory and learning and age and various outcome measures (Chap. 1).
- Knowledge of evidence-based practice: how to create knowledge/evidence and how to evaluate and apply relevant evidence, generally and to individual older people. That is, implementation science or knowledge translation (how to bridge the gap between knowledge and practice) .
- Expertise in promoting and 'selling' a product most people do not want to buy—diabetes!
- Expertise in change management—ability to change themselves and help older people with diabetes and often families understand and make relevant changes.
- To be generally literate as well as health literate and the ability to assess health literacy in others.
- To understand how to evaluate the care they provide and select care outcomes relevant to the older individual rather than just using patient reported outcome measures (PROM), patient satisfaction and HbA1c. That is thoughtful personalised assessment to match the personalised care plan. Such assessment might include using patient-generated tools (Jenkinson and McGee 1998).
- To understand the importance of economic evaluation and demonstrate how the HP and the service add value to the whole.
- To be able to work with and within multidisciplinary teams in order to support people with chronic diseases, provide integrated care and streamline care transitions (Brownie et al. 2014).
- The courage to evaluate their performance (fit for purpose) and/or/be evaluated by colleagues and older people with diabetes.

3.8 Theory of Mind

The ability to understand older individuals with diabetes is a crucial skill that enables complex relationships to develop. Thus, HPs need a well-developed Theory of Mind (TOM). TOM is a set of attributes that enables humans (and other great apes) to reason about another person's thoughts. It is not a single ability: it is a collection of empathy, taking a perspectives and appreciation intent and is considered to be the hallmark of rich cognition (Keim 2017).

HPs with well-developed TOM are more skilled at managing complex social relationships and diverse people such as older people with diabetes in health care settings. Researchers distinguish between effective and cognitive TOM. Effective TOM applies to the ability to identify one's own and other people's emotions, which is positively linked to empathy and negatively to antisocial behaviours (Shamay-Tsoory et al. 2010). Cognitive TOM is concerned with inferences and representations of other people's beliefs and intentions.

A growing body of evidence suggests reading literary fiction enhances self-reported empathy and understanding of other people's lives, possibly because it is an active process and 'forces' the reader to engage with the characters in the book: that is, to engage in TOM (Kidd and Castano 2013). It can also be a component and an outcome of qualitative research (Furman 2007).

Reading fiction might also challenge reader's expectations and thinking because readers use their own experience and explanatory models to understand the characters in the book, fill in gaps and search for meaning in the various possible meanings—just like finding meaning in people's health care stories with their clues and cues. HPs have to explore the clues and stories with the individual to understand the meaning in the story. Therefore, it is possible that reading literary fiction be an unacknowledged core HP competency and a key aspect of communication. Table 3.1 outlines some benefits of reading literary fiction and Box 3.1 lists some literary fiction books.

Box 3.1: Some Recommended Literary Fiction HPs Could Read to Improve Theory of Mind

Cameron B. (2010) A Dog's Purpose Pan McMillan, New York.

Chekov A. (2003) Chekov's Doctors: a Collection of Medical Tales. Kent State University, Kent Ohio.

Chekov A. (1984) The Doctor translated by Garnett C ECCO, New York.

Ogawa (2003) The Housekeeper and the Professor Translated by Snyder S, Picador Press.

Shakespeare W. The Collected Works.

Hawk E. (2015) Rules for a Knight. Hutchinson, London.

Lazarus J. (2016) *Listen Like a Dog and Make a Difference in the World* HCI Books, Deerfield Beach.

Wong S-M. (2012) Translated by Kim K-Y. The Dog Who Dared to Dream. Abercus, London.

Pasternak B. (1957) Doctor Zhivago Gianiacomo Feltrinelli Publisher Italy.

Williams M. The Velveteen Rabbit. GH Doran Publisher Company New York.

White TH. (1958) The Once and Future King. Collins, London.

Blyton E. (1944) The Magic Faraway Tree. Hardie Grant.

3.9   Metaphors

The greatest thing by far is to be the master of the metaphor (Aristotle 384–322)

Table 3.1 Some postulated benefits of reading literary fiction derived from studies undertaken by psychologists and based on information in Kidd and Castano (2013), Seiter (2015), Wilson et al. (2013), and Vemuri and Mormino (2013)

Benefit	Possible mechanism for the benefit
Empathy and understanding	MRI studies show imagining stories activates the regions of the brain concerned with interactions with other people, especially when trying to understand their thoughts and feelings
	The brain's capacity to construct a map of other people's intentions is referred to as Theory of Mind (TOM). Stories/narrative medicine enables HPs to engage TOM
Stress-management/ disengagement	Periods of disengagement are important to prevent cognitive overload and reduce cognitive function. Reading fiction helps people disengage. Regular readers report less stress, better sleep, higher self-esteem and less depression than non-readers. Reading for short periods reduces stress by 60% (slower heart rate, les muscle tension and quieter mind) more than listening to music, drinking tea, walking and playing video games
Improve sleep	Relaxation helps sleep especially if combined with a sleep ritual. Reading non-fiction encourages projection into the future compared to reading fiction
Improve relationships	Reading produces a type of 'reality simulation' similar to computer simulations that help understand complex situations and relationships. Science fiction that concerns the future helps people understand change and that they can cope with the change
Maintain memory	Readers have slower memory changes in later life compared to non-reader peers, and show fewer characteristics of Alzheimer's disease
Open-minded	Reading pages about discrimination from Harry Potter books suggests attitudes can change. It is not clear whether the change is short term of loner lasting
Improve creativity	Fiction is more ambiguous than most movies, which encourages creativity and processing information
Build vocabulary	Readers show more activity in the areas of the brain associated with understanding language, especially the left temporal cortex
	You can check vocabulary ontestyourvocab.com
Benefit research	Qualitative data analysis can be enhanced by reading literary fiction, which can aid the researchers to find meaning and purposes in interview and other data
	It can be doubly meaningful if the data is co-analysed with the informants, e.g. through member checking
	It helps reduce the power imbalance in research and change from research into people to doing research with them
	It enhances the credibility of the research, its authenticity and applicability outside the sample population
	Significantly, it helps the reader experience the phenomena

The original Greek meaning of metaphor is to 'carry something across' or 'transfer'. In the context of this chapter metaphor refers to the way older people with diabetes transfer their health stories and the way HPs transfer information to older people with diabetes. People use an average of three metaphors per 100 words. Metaphors enliven language, even HP language: they are interactive, engage, develop problem-solving skills, create outcome possibilities and encourage autonomous decision-making.

In health care, metaphors can be generated by older people with diabetes, HPs or collaboratively. For example:

Person with diabetes: *I've reached the end of the road now I end insulin.*

HP: *Insulin is not the end of the road.*

What is the end of the road? For the person with diabetes it meant insulin is her last treatment option. The end of the road is death. Did the HP recognise the metaphor?

Collaborative metaphors are constructed together to meet the individual's needs using shared decision-making strategies (Chap. 2).

*That doctor said I **have** to start insulin. He says that every time I come—so I usually ignore him or I don't come.*

I will not start insulin.

The doctors' referral note highlighted Mrs. TZ's very high HbA1c, over 9%, her complications, her 'psychological insulin resistance', and her low health and general literacy.

How about we have a chat so we can get to know each other and you can tell me a little about yourself?

Ok. I live over there in the park. It's not very nice and the doctor told me I had to keep my insulin in the fridge—what fridge. No fidges in the park.

What if we could keep the insulin cool another way?

I remember my foster father used to keep his beer cold in the river. But there is no river in the park, just a very dirty lake and a basin in the toilet.

Mrs. TZ's low literacy did not prevent her from thinking creatively and apply past experience to the current issue. Maybe her psychological insulin resistance was actually a practical problem.

My dad used to do that too when he went fishing.

OK. I'm going now. I will think about the insulin.

I received a letter from Mrs. TZ 2 days later. I read that letter very carefully looking for meaning and purpose in her words and clues to how I could help her. I felt the letter was a test. If I passed the test we had the basis for a relationship. If I failed I would be just another unhelpful HP.

I received many long rambling letters from Mrs. TZ over the years. Each letter was a test. I had to try to identify what she wanted to talk about from the information she provided. Over time she shared her story of sexual abuse, using illicit drugs and many succeeded attempts. She was regularly referred for psychiatric appointments but she did not keep many—most were with male psychiatrists.

3.10 Expressive Writing and Health

Mrs. TZ's letters are a form of expressive writing. Expressive writing or therapeutic writing can be used in a number of ways to achieve therapeutic goals such as to relieve stress and to find meaning in and understand the disease and the emotions it evokes. There are many examples of such writing including HP's writing about facing death and other stressful life events. Expressive writing is also used in aged care homes to document people's life history and help them remember as their cognition changes. The diary of Anne Frank is one of the best known examples of expressive writing: she said:

> ...*the brightest spot of all is that at least I can write down all my thoughts and feelings, otherwise I'd absolutely suffocate* (Anne Frank, March 16 1944)

3.11 Cultural Competence

For the purposes of this chapter 'culture' refers to the person's ethnicity. However, culture embodies a great deal more than ethnicity and the country the individual was born in. It also encompasses factors such as workplace culture; health care is also a particular culture with its language and traditions. Lessons and habits acquired from others such as parents and peers cluster among populations and regions (Keim 2017).

Migration from one country (the home country) to another country occurs through choice and through displacement due to wars and natural disasters. Migration is a global phenomenon: one in 30 individuals in the world is a migrant (Future Capacity 2014). Many migrants are older people who come alone, join family in the new country or have family join them.

The culture and language is often very different in the new country. Interpreters are often required in health setting and everyday life. Consequently, HPs need to understand the issues older migrants face, often many years after they actually migrated.

Misunderstanding can occur through inappropriate communication, which can undermine trust and personalised care and increase the risk of adverse events and errors (Hadziabdic et al. (2015). Interpreting services can help address the communication issues, provided services are accessible when needed. However, consultations with interpreters present change the dynamics of the consultation. Three main types of interpreter are described:

1. Professional interpreters who are trained to interpret, and medical and cultural competence and can be accessed in person or by telephone.
2. Informal interpreters, often relatives of all ages, friends and bilingual staff employees who usually do not have any relevant training and may not have the required health literacy skills.
3. Bilingual HPs of all disciplines (PASS International 2008).

Important ethical issues such as privacy and confidentiality, gender issues such as husbands speaking for their wives in some cultures and coercion can arise and HPs need to know how to manage these issues as well as the actual communication process.

Consultations are influenced by the situation, the issues being discussed, the individual, the HP and the interpreter. Satisfactory interpretation occurs when messages are conveyed as accurately as possible. That might not be word-for-word (Dysart-Gale et al. 2007) as many HPs expect because there might not be an exact translation.

Sleptsova et al. (2017) used Roter Interaction Analysis (RIAS) to analyse 19 video recordings of interpreted consultations between HPs and 'patients'. They identified significant differences in the number of utterances in the original language compared with the target language. Approximately 33% of HP's utterances were not translated. The interpreters did not explain the omitted information to the HP or the patient.

Another study explored the issues that could affect interpreter-mediated medical consultations and perceptions of interpreters by observing 20 consultations with people from a range of ethnic backgrounds followed by semi-structured interviews (Ra 2017). Interpreters report challenges in discussions concerning end of life situations, that involve family members, when patients did not ask questions and interpreting non-verbal communication. They indicated having relevant information before consultations, adequate time, and HPs having realistic expectations of the interpreter's role could help.

Understanding people's cultural beliefs is important. For example, Abdoli et al. (2011) found Iranian people living in Iran regarded their doctor as an Imam (Holy Man) and placed significant faith in the doctor and his or her decisions and felt empowered by their doctor, despite not actively participating in care planning. Their religious beliefs helped them manage their diabetes, even though they attributed diabetes to God's Will or fate. They felt they had a responsibility to look after themselves because their body was a gift from God.

The ability to deliver culturally appropriate care can be enhanced through training programmes using community-based participatory approaches (McElfish 2017). The programme improved cultural knowledge, competence and performance and the organisations that participated made policy and environmental changes. HPs' and other worker's ability to deliver culturally appropriate care can be enhanced through training programmes using community-based participatory approaches (McElfish 2017).

Immigrant people often meet in 'gossip groups' to exchange stories, validate their own and other people's experiences and share information. These stories underscore commonalities among the group, the insider view, and help people manage in their new country (Manderson and Allotey 2003).

3.12   Dignity

Dignity is a complex multifaceted concept and is greater than the notion of being human. Some humans think they have a right to dignity because they are human. Actually there is no agreed definition of what dignity actually means (Clark 2010). The word is derived from the Latin *dignus* meaning worthy of honour or respect, which suggests people needs to have certain attributes to attain *dignus*.

As an objective concept, dignity is the basis for human rights where it is a value. Subjectively, dignity can be experienced and enables individual differences to be considered. Dignity encompasses self-regarding and other-regarding dignity (Gallagher 2004). Gallagher (2004) proposed nurses should consider dignity from both perspectives. Dignity is also culturally dependent. It is learned through sociali- sation and social and cultural norms. Dignity may be present, it can be lost and/or the factors that contribute to a person's dignity discounted.

The following anecdote shows dignity does not depend on independence but it might depend on self-concept and enhance self-efficacy. The anecdote is also an example of other-regarded dignity, insensitivity and disrespect, as well as ageism. The woman's families' dignity would have been compromised if they overheard the conversation and could have resulted in a complaint and reprimand for the staff members concerned.

Look at her! All contracted and skinny, with pressure ulcers everywhere.

Yeah—I do not know why she has her hair done every week and her nails—she 85!!

I know. And look at all her dresses hanging in the wardrobe—what that for, she can't wear them now.

She gets upset if she can't see them though. Bit of a waste if you ask me.

'She' was an old lady living in an aged care home. It had been her home for over 5 years.

'They' were care assistants who assisted her with routine Activities of Daily Living ADLs, including getting ready for the hairdresser and manicurist.

'She' migrated from the UK after World War 2 when she was in her late 20s. She worked for 'Bomber Command' during the War flying newly made bomber aero- planes from they were manufacturer to the airfields from whence pilots flew them to bomb the enemy. She was always immaculately dressed. Her dresses and beauty routine were a key part of her personal dignity.

HPs need to consider ways of maintaining older people with diabetes, and their families' dignity understood as autonomy, self-respect and self-worth. They can:

- Affirm the individual's personhood.
- Acknowledge that people are profoundly affected by how others see them as well as how they see themselves.
- Emphasise that having diabetes, being old and changed function should not diminish their dignity.
- Value them as a person with a story, relationships, and dreams and hopes.

The inability to acknowledge personhood—the insensitivity of not acknowledging person- hood - can be psychologically devastating (Chochinov 2016)

3.13   Summary

Chapter 3 aimed to be proactive and present new ways of considering HP knowledge and competence and suggest ways HP skills, attitudes and beliefs enhance or detract from shared decision-making and personalised care.

The authors invite HPs to use quantum thinking—look at themselves and their roles in new ways to use 'dialogue education'. Dialogue education is informed by quantum thinking and its core concepts: relatedness, a holistic perspective, duality, uncertainty, participation and energy. These concepts are at the heart of personalised care and shared decision-making.

3.14   Reflection Points

1. Reflect on the quote on Page xx beginning 'Perdu collected the words...' and consider
   (a) How the quote applies to personalising care with older people with diabetes?
   (b) What is Perdu referring to when he mentions 'the soul?'
   (c) How could you penetrate 'the fog of words' to find out what a person with diabetes might not choose to reveal.
   (d) How could you clarify your assumptions about the 'fog?'
2. Most HPs use some form of reflective practice knowingly or subconsciously. Theoretically, reflection could help older people understand their behaviours and diabetes. How could you help older people with diabetes use reflection to understand themselves, their diabetes and their health status to enhance their confidence to self-care?
3. Think about the anecdote describing personal dignity. What would you do if you overheard the care assistants' conversation? Did they acknowledge the woman's personhood?

References

Abdoli S, Ashktorab T, Ahmadi F et al (2011) Religion, faith and the empowerment process: stories of Iranian people with diabetes. Int J Nurs Pract 17:289–298

Acosta A, Douthwaite B (2005) Appreciative Inquiry—an approach for learning and change based on our best practice. Manner of Things, pp 1–4

Arias-Carballal M (2017) A teacher's personal-emotional identity and its reflection upon the development of his professional identity. Qual Rep 22(6):1693–1709

Asal J-P, Assal T (2013) Role of creative arts in diabetes care. In: Dunning T (ed) Diabetes education: art, science and evidence. Wiley Blackwell, Chichester, pp 98–116

Barabino B, Malavia M, Assal J-P (2009) Art beyond therapy: when patients and healthcare providers share the limelight. Diabetes Voice 54:36–39

Bombeke K, Van Roosbroeck S, De Winter B et al (2011) Medical students trained in communication skills show a decline in patient-centred attitudes: an observational study comparing two cohorts during clinical clerkships. Patient Educ Couns 84(3):310–318

Brownie S, Thomas J, McAllister L, Groves M (2014) Australian health reforms: enhancing interprofessional practice and competency within the workforce. J Interprof Care 28(3):252–253

Chochinov H (2016) How to uphold patient dignity at the end of life. palliativecare.org.au/.../how-to-upload-patient-dignity-at-end-of-life

Chopra D (undated) https://www.google.com.au/url?url=https://www.deepakchopra.com/blog/article/4361&rct=j&frm=1&q=&esrc=s&sa=U&ved=0ahUKEwjHvISv9efXAhUFnZQKHaluDRsQFggWMAA&usg=AOvVaw0YgW9F5HfsPhD4oW0DgOh1957

Choudhry N, Fletcher R (2006) Systematic review: the relationship between clinical experience and quality of health care. Ann Intern Med 142:260–273

Clark J (2010) Defining the concept of dignity and developing a model to promote its use in practice. Nursing Times. https://www.nursingtimes.net/roles/practice-nurses/defining-the-concept-of-dignity

Dysart-Gale D (2007) Clinicians and medical interpreters: negotiating culturally appropriate care for patients with limited English ability. Fam Community Health 30(3):237–246

Einstein A (1879–1955) https://www.goodreads.com/.../253933-i-never-teach-my-pupils-i-only-attempt-to-provide

Father Brown The Grim Reaper (2014) (TV Episode) Accessed via: Quotes - IMDb www.imdb.com/title/tt3445568/quotes

Furman R (2007) Poetry narrative as qualitative data: explorations into existential theory. Indo-Pac J Phenomenol 7(1):1–21

Future capacity needs in managing health aspects of migration. http://publications.iom.int/bookstore/free/WMR_capicity_needs_health_aspects.pdf

Gallagher A (2004) Dignity and respect for dignity—two key health professional values: implications for nursing practice. Nurs Ethics 11, 587–599

George N (2015) The Little Paris Bookshop. Little Brown Book Company, London

Hadziabdic E, Lundin C, Hjelm K (2015) BMC Health Serv 15:458. https://doi.org/10.1186/s12913=015-1124-5

Haight B, Christ M, Dias J (1994) Does nursing education promote ageism? J Adv Nurs 20(20):382–390

Hickey J, Newhouse R, Koithan M, et al (2013) Credentialling; the need for a national research agenda. ScienceDirect. https://doi.org/10.1016/outlook.2013.10.001

Hoff B (1982) The Tao of Pooh. Dutton Books, New York

Jenkinson C, McGee H (1998) Health status measurement. Radcliff Medical Press, Oxford

Keim B (2017) Animal minds: what they think, feel and know. National Geographic, New York, pp 95–100

Kidd D, Castano E (2013) Reading literary fiction improves theory of mind. Science express. http://www.sciencemag.org/content/early/recent/3 October 2013/page 1/10.1126/science.1239918

King A, Hoppe R (2013) 'Best practice' for patient-centered communication: a narrative review. J Grad Med Educ 5(3):385–393

Lacey S (2013) https://www.theguardian.com/...culture.../harry-seidler-architecture

Langewitz W, Denz M, Keller A, Kiss A, Rüttimann S, Wössmer B. Spontaneous talking time at start of consultation in outpatient clinic: cohort study. BMJ 2002; 325: 682–683

Lazarus J (2016) Listen like a dog and make your mark on the world. Health Communications Inc, Deerfield Beach

Lothian K, Philip I (2001) Maintaining the dignity and autonomy of older people in the health care setting. Br Med J 322(287):668–670

Manderson L, Allotey P (2003) Storytelling, marginality, and community in Australia: how immigrants position their difference in health care settings. Med Anthropol 20:1–21

Mann K, Gordon J, MacLeod A (2009) Reflection and reflective practice in health professions education: a systematic review. Adv Health Sci Educ 14:595–521

McElfiish P (2017) Evaluation of a multicomponent cultural competency training program, Arkanal, 2015–2016. Res Chronic Dis 14(6):E62

Nam S, Chesla C, Stotts N et al (2011) Barriers to diabetes management: patient and provider factors. Diabetes Res Clin Pract 93(1):1–9

PASS International v.z.w (2008) Is the use of interpreters in medical consultations justified? A critical review of the literature. www.pass-international.org

Ra S (2017) Intercultural communication: challenges in interpreter-mediated medical consultations AUSIT In Touch Magazine. Vol 25 #1. http://ausit.org/AUSIT/Publications/Newsletter/AUSIT/Publications/Newsletter.aspx

Seiter (2015) https://open.buffer.com/reading.fiction/

Shamay-Tsoory S, Harari H, Aharon-Peretz J (2010) The role of the orbitofrontal cortex in affective theory of mind deficits in criminal offenders with psychopathic tendencies. Cortex 46:668–667

Sleptsova M, Weber H, Schopf A (2017) Using interpreters in medical consultations: what I said and what is translated—a descriptive analysis using RIAS. J Patient Educ Couns 100:1667. https://doi.org/10.1016/jpec.2017.03.023

Vemuri P, Mormino E (2013) Cognitive stimulating activities to keep dementia at bay. Neurology 81:308

Weiner S, Schwartz A, Sharma G et al (2013) Patient-centered decision-making and health care outcomes: an observational study. Ann Intern Med 158(8):573–579

Wilson R, Boyle P, Yu L et al (2013) Life-span cognitive activity, neuropathologic burden, and cognitive aging. Neurology 81:314

Yassin T (1994) Exacerbation of a perennial problem? The theory-practice gap and changes in nurse education. Prof Nurse 10:183–187

From Research to Evidence to Context: Implementing and Using Guidelines as Decision Aids to Personalise Care

Trisha Dunning

I have been impressed with the urgency of doing. Knowing is not enough. We must apply.

(Leonardo da Vinci 1452)

Key Points

- Clinical guidelines represent the distillation of available evidence into recommendations—they are essentially a form of consensus.
- Guidelines may not address important contextual issues for organisations or individuals.
- Guidelines must be contextualised to relevant organisations, clinical situations and individual older people with diabetes to be useful.
- Unless we ask the 'right' questions we are likely to miss contextual and other issues that are essential to personalised care.
- It is necessary to identify the unique elements of an organisation or an individual's life to consider context.
- The Knowledge to Action framework can be used to implement guidelines in most practice settings/organisational context. Shared decision-making can help identify the person's unique context.

Diabetes does not define me or my life and often it is not the issue I am coming to see you about.

T. Dunning, A.M., M.Ed., Ph.D., R.N., C.D.E.
Centre for Quality and Patient Safety Research, Barwon Health Partnership,
Deakin University, Geelong, VIC, Australia
e-mail: trisha.dunning@barwonhealth.org.au;
trisha.dunning@deakin.edu.au

© Springer International Publishing AG, part of Springer Nature 2018
T. Dunning (ed.), *The Art and Science of Personalising Care with Older People with Diabetes*, https://doi.org/10.1007/978-3-319-74360-8_4

4.1   Introduction

Guidelines are a key part of integrated diabetes care. However, they are often not implemented effectively, or used, for a range of reasons (Turner et al. 2008). They are more likely to be used if key HP, other end users, and care recipients, in this case people with diabetes, are involved in the development and implementation processes. Box 4.1 shows a list of commonly used 'diabetes guidelines'.

Caring for older people with diabetes becomes more challenging with long duration of diabetes and as function and life expectancy change. Most guidelines concerning the care of older people with diabetes are based on the best available evidence. However, there is very little randomised control trial evidence to support many recommendations because many older people with diabetes do not meet the 'exclusionary' inclusion criteria (Bayer Tadd 2006), see Chap. 10. Thus, many recommendations concerning older people with diabetes represent expert consensus opinion. For example, The International Diabetes Federation (IDF) Global Guideline for Managing Type 2 Diabetes (2013) and The McKellar Guidelines (Dunning et al. 2013a).

Box 4.1: Some Examples of 'Diabetes Guidelines'
American Diabetes Association (ADA). *Standards of medical care in diabetes—2017.* care.diabetesjournals.org/content/diacare/suppl/.../DC_40_S1_final.pdf

Royal Australian College General Practitioners- General practice management of type 2 diabetes. www.racgp.org.au/your-practice/guidelines/diabetes/

Best practice guidelines—Diabetes Australia. https://www.diabetesaustralia.com.au/best-practice-guidelines

National Institute of Clinical Excellence (NICE). Type 2 diabetes in adults: management|Guidance. https://www.nice.org.uk/guidance/ng28

Type 1 diabetes in adults: diagnosis and management—NICE. https://www.nice.org.uk/guidance/ng17

Scottish Intercollegiate Guideline Network (SIGN). SIGN 116 Management of diabetes. www.sign.ac.uk/sign-116-management-of-diabetes.html

Beers List: Potentially Inappropriate Drugs for Elderly—MPR. www.empr.com/clinical-charts/beers-list-potentially.../125908/

STOPP/START criteria for potentially inappropriate ...—NCBI—NIH. https://www.ncbi.nlm.nih.gov/pmc/articles/PMC4339726/

The McKellar Guidelines for Managing Older People with Diabetes. https://www.adma.org.au/.../133-the-mckellar-guidelines-for-managing-older-people-with-diabetes-in-residential-and-other-care-settings_

All guidelines, including consensus-based guidelines, need to be developed using recommended guideline development processes. Their consensus status does not necessarily represent inferior quality, given they are based on the best available evidence; they have the added benefit of clinical experience. It is imperative that guideline recommendations make 'clinical sense' and that the content, language and design meet the needs of the HPs who will use them. Although there is a great deal of information available about identifying, grading and synthesising evidence guidance, relatively little attention is paid to the design features that enhance readability and appeal of the final guidelines, which could be one reason they are not used.

For example, the design and layout of The McKellar Guidelines was given as much attention as the content, when they were developed. Design emerged as a key factor in their highly rated acceptability to end users during the evaluation phase. However, when they were implemented as policy in one organisation where they were tested, they had to be redesigned to conform to the electronic format required for organisational policies. Staff frequently request hard copies because the electronic format is 'ugly and hard to follow'. More about The McKellar Guidelines later.

The content must be relevant to specific situations in which older people with diabetes receive care, and address their health issues, not just their diabetes. Care must be integrated and focused on healthy ageing and personalised care to 'preserve function to enable well-being', given people aged 60 and older are at increased risk of chronic disease, frailty and care dependency (World Health Organisation (WHO) 2017a, b, c).

Although many recent 'diabetes clinical guidelines' recommend personalising care, they largely focus on diabetes outcomes and metabolic targets, rather than other aspects of care. Likewise, most do not indicate how the guidelines can be used in practice, refer to other relevant guidelines, or make recommendations about important general health care issue that need to be considered in the individual's overall care plan.

Some HPs do not have the knowledge or training to recognise functional and geriatric syndromes. Signs and symptoms are often atypical or are masked in older people, which is often not reflected in guidelines and other care documents such as hypoglycaemia management. Likewise, a great deal of undergraduate and postgraduate diabetes education still focuses on 'textbook' signs and symptoms, which means key health issues can be missed or delayed, for example, delirium, hypoglycaemia and myocardial infarction.

The key to implementing guidelines and using them to personalise care for individuals depends on exemplary communication, sound clinical reasoning and informed decision-making (Chaps. 2 and 3). Communication is challenging when older people have sensory deficits such as sight and hearing, are unwell, or have cognitive changes and when other people such as family and interpreters are present. Hypo- and hyperglycaemia can affect cognition in the short term. It is also challenging to determine what is clinically relevant from an individual's story, yet interpreting people's stories is vital to personalised care, see Chap. 3.

4.2   Clinical Decision-Making: The Art of Combining Qualitative and Quantitative Information

Clinical decision-making involves:

- Making a diagnosis from the person's story, their signs and symptoms and a comprehensive assessment.
- Matching the diagnosis with the best evidence (guideline recommendations). Many HPs stop at that step and decide management (Weiner 2004).
- Discussing the diagnosis and care options, their implications and risks and benefits with the individual and/or family, if relevant, to fit the evidence to the individual and not the individual to the research. This step might involve using decision aids and/or conducting a case conference.
- Using 'choice' language and 'options' language and knowing when to use decision language. Language is important to shared decision-making (Chap. 2).
- A collaborative endeavour to reach a shared decision where the HP accepting the person's decision. The insider view (person with diabetes) and outsider view (HP) are likely to differ.

Finding out people's stories and undertaking an assessment yields many pieces of a jigsaw puzzle.

Clinical reasoning is the process of putting the pieces together to form a picture.

The picture helps shared decision-making.

HPs need self-knowledge, sensitivity and reflexivity to engage in personalised clinical reasoning and decision-making. Reflexivity refers to systematically reflecting on how knowledge and behaviours are constructed and being aware of how the HP's personal beliefs, experiences, values and biases shape their actions (Malterud 2001). Reflexivity might be particularly important to HPs who have diabetes themselves.

Reflexivity is a core aspect of rigour in qualitative research. Researchers reflect in and on their potential influence on the research, including participants and the overall outcomes throughout a study, and document them in field notes. A similar process can be used in clinical situations although the reflections might not be formally documented. Clinical decision-making also relies on a great deal of qualitative data—the individual's story.

Significantly, personalised care is determined by the relationship between the older person and the HP, including the HP's ability to recognise the individual's health concerns at the time and the way they see and experience them (Starfield 2011). Good relationships lead to 'healing'. Healing refers to the Anglo Saxon concept of 'haelan', to make whole (Modern English-Old English Dictionary 2017). It encompasses spiritual and physical health and connectedness.

4.3   Guidelines

Guidelines are resources that can help HPs decide care with older people with diabetes/families. Guidelines also highlight the education and training issues HPs might require (Corriere et al. 2014). In some countries, the use of guidelines and clinical algorithms is linked to funding and payment for performance. Funding is provided for chronic disease management and other activities. It is rarely provided for communication skills or for paying attention to an individual's defined problems or solutions (Starfield 2011) because they can predispose HPs to focus on the disease, in this care diabetes.

Most Guidelines are evidenced based, but the evidence is largely based on results derived from groups of highly selected individuals who may be very different from the older people the HP cares for. This is a form of selection bias and is described in Chap. 10. Likewise, outcome measures that attract reimbursement might not be suitable for the safety of many older people, e.g. HbA1c <7% for an older person on insulin who eats erratically and is cognitively impaired, see Chap. 1. Guideline can be used as decision aids or be used to develop decision aids.

4.4   Decision Aids

Decision aids are evidence-based tools designed to help people and HPs participate in choosing management strategies from various options. Decision aids vary in format and detail and can be interactive or static, electronic or paper based, but generally outline:

- The decision/s to be considered.
- Evidence-based information about the disease/health issue.
- Available options.
- The benefits and risks of each option.
- Scientific uncertainties.

Decision aids improve communication, help people think about their options, weight up the information (evidence) and uncertainties and make a choice (Chapman 2017; Stacey et al. 2009). People may actually need time to read and reflect on the information, especially older people. At present very few, if any, diabetes-related decision aids are available. The author is currently developing a suite of information (decision aids) for older people with diabetes, their families and HPs to help them initiate conversations about palliative and end of life diabetes care. They are currently being evaluated. Importantly, the key writing group includes older people with diabetes and their advice and experience is invaluable and irreplaceable.

The effectiveness of decision aids is influenced by the individual's health at the time and their decisional capacity, preferences and psychological distance. Psychological distance, a construct derived from construal theory, refers to the extent to which an individual 'removes' themselves from others (Nugent Pam 2013), which in turn influences people's thinking about issues such as other people, interventions and technology (Trope and Liberman 2010). It applies to HPs and older people with diabetes.

Psychological distance can be temporal, social, spatial or hypothetical (Trope and Liberman 2010). Decisions can be concrete or abstract, depending on psychological distance. Thinking about more distant events such as future complications evokes abstract thinking. Thinking about events close to the time evokes more concrete thinking. Thus, the further away the event is, the easier it is to make abstract considered decisions. Psychological distance influences decisions and could be one reason people change their mind over time as events get closer, e.g. end of life .

Although older people with diabetes value being involved in care decisions and shared decision-making leads to improved outcomes (Carmen et al. 2013), it is not always possible. Shared decision-making occurs on three levels:

1. Micro level—decisions are shared
2. Meso level—evidence-based medicine for specific populations often distilled in guidelines and decision aids
3. Macro level—public preferences and regulatory frameworks.

Several frameworks for developing interventions and policies to support patient and family engagement are available and most are multidimensional (Carmen et al. 2013). Multidimensional engagement includes:

- Older people with diabetes and families—preferences, all stages of the research process from identifying issues to deigning and conducting research (Harris et al. 2015).
- Direct care providers—evidence of what is needed and what works.
- Researchers—provide evidence.
- Organisations—design and governance.
- Policy makers—systems and implementation strategies.

4.5   Knowledge Translation: Implementing Guidelines and Decision Aids

Applying evidence in practice is often slow, which means people may not be offered treatment or receive treatment they do not need or is outdated and may be unsafe (Graham et al. 2006). For example, using 'top up/stat doses of insulin to correct isolated episodes of hyperglycaemia in aged care homes. Even when guidelines are effectively disseminated or implemented, they are often not used as the guideline developers intended (Grenhalghh et al. 2004).

Several 'knowledge implementation frameworks' exist and the barriers are well described and have not changed over time. Barriers related to the characteristics of the intervention, the situation/context of the target audience, and research reporting the intervention including sample limitations on economic evaluation (Glasgow and

Emmons 2007). Some of these barriers suggest the intervention/guidelines might not address the needs of or context in which they will be used (Green et al. 2009).

Knowledge translation encompasses:

- Turning knowledge into action through creating and applying knowledge/ evidence.
- Continuing education based on the best available evidence in all forms including guidelines and could include improving research engagement.
- Engaging with key stakeholders at the knowledge development stage where possible (Green et al. 2009; Graham et al. 2006).

The next section describes to illustrate the way guideline development recommendations and translation strategies were used to develop, evaluate and implement The McKellar Guidelines and ultimately improve the care of older people with diabetes.

4.6   The McKellar Guidelines

The McKellar Guidelines are unique, in that they advocate for personalised care, were developed in close collaboration with the multidisciplinary clinicians who would use them and were implemented in a range of aged care settings to evaluate their impact on practice as well as their usability, acceptance and clinical relevance before they were placed in the public domain. Older people with diabetes and family members participated in the evaluation (Dunning et al. 2013a). The final Guideline consists of 18 individual care issues and five risk assessment tools, see Table 4.1.

The topics for the 18 care issues were decided with clinicians who care for older people with diabetes. Each individual topic/guideline includes three sections:

- Care context—why do it
- Assessment—what to look for
- Care planning—how to plan care

The Guidelines are underpinned by a proactive, risk identification/minimisation approach to each older person's care. They were designed to be used with other relevant guidelines, policies and screening tools and to benchmark the quality of care of older people with diabetes. This process helped HPs consider the multimorbidity context of caring for most older people with diabetes because they are not only 'diabetes focused'.

4.7   The Process Used to Develop The McKellar Guidelines

The McKellar Guidelines were developed using *The National Health and Medical Research Council Guidelines for Developing Clinical Guidelines* (NHMRC 1995) and the *WHO Handbook of Guideline Development* (2017), which consist of:

Table 4.1 The 18 individual topic/care issues and the five risk assessment tools addressed in The McKellar Guidelines

Individual topics/issues
1. Consulting with the General Practitioner (GP)
2. Admission Assessment and Diabetes Risk Screening
(a) Residents not Known to Have Diabetes
(b) Residents with Diabetes
3. Blood Glucose Monitoring
4. Hyperglycaemia and Sick Day Management
5. Hypoglycaemia
6. Managing Glucose Lowering Medicines
7. Managing Corticosteroid (Steroids) and Antipsychotic Medicines
8. RACF Annual Diabetes Health Assessment (Annual Cycle of Care)
9. Diabetes-specific Falls risk
10. Pain Associated with Diabetes
11. Foot Care
12. Nutrition and Hydration
13. Oral Health Care
14. Well-being, Quality of Life and Depression
15. Palliative and End of Life Care
16. Cognitive Impairment and Dementia
17. Sexual Health and Well-Being
18. Managing a Disaster if RACF is Affected
Risk assessment tools
1. Diabetes risk
2. Hypoglycaemia
3. Diabetes-specific pain
4. Diabetes-specific falls risk factors
5. Medicine-related adverse events

- Establishing an interdisciplinary health professional expert advisory group, which consisted of nurses, geriatricians, general practitioners, pharmacists and personal care workers to provide feedback about the content, design and layout of successive iterations of the Guidelines.
- Declaring conflicts of interest.
- Identifying and synthesising the best available evidence using a structured literature review and narrative synthesis.
- Formulating the guidelines and associated recommendations. This was an iterative approach where several iterations were developed, discussed with the expert advisory group and modified as needed.
- Implementing the draft guidelines in large and small aged care facilities and community aged care in metropolitan, regional and rural areas in small group workshops and evaluating their use in practice over 9–12 months.
- Undertaking interviews with HPs using the guidelines. Targeted focus groups with relevant experts and interviewing older people with diabetes where HPs used the guidelines to plan care.

- Subjecting the Guideline to independent external peer review.
- Finalising and releasing the Guideline.

This collaborative process enabled care issues of concern to a wide range of HPs to be identified and addressed and enhanced the clinical relevance and usefulness of the final Guideline.

4.8   The Knowledge-to-Action Framework

The Knowledge-to-Action framework consists of two main components but each component has several overlapping phases:

1. Knowledge/evidence creation; in this care The McKellar Guidelines.
2. An Action cycle, to identify the actions needed to adapt the knowledge/evidence (McKellar Guidelines) to particular settings, apply the knowledge to practice and monitor the outcomes (Graham 2006; Field et al. 2014).

The action cycle included the implementation process, which starts by deciding the rationale for using The Guidelines and developing a process for managing any changes required to current practice by collaboratively deciding what facilitators and barriers exist in the particular practice setting, how to manage them, and what evaluation process will be used to assess outcomes. Appointing a designated 'champion' and supporting them to perform the role is more likely to result in successful implementation than *an* ad hoc process (Kadu and Stolee 2015).

The care plans of older people with diabetes were evaluated before and approximately nine months after The McKellar Guidelines were implemented in a large regional aged care homes and four small rural community-based aged care homes by auditing medical record to determine whether The Guidelines were used to plan care. In addition, HPs and people with diabetes and families were interviewed about their experiences.

An outcome of the HP interviews was a recommendation to provide specific suggestions about how The Guidelines could be used. Consequently, *The McKellar Way* (Dunning et al. 2013b) was developed as a companion to The Guidelines. The outcomes and impact of the Guidelines have been monitored as much as possible since their release in late 2013 and are the outcomes are shown in Table 4.2.

4.9   The McKellar Guidelines and the Knowledge-to-Action Framework

The Knowledge-to-Action framework was a useful way of implementing The McKellar Guidelines in the study settings and subsequently in several practice setting. In addition, *The McKellar Way: How to Use The McKellar Guidelines* can help HPs become familiar with The Guideline. It provides some specific, practical

Table 4.2 Main outcomes and impact of The McKellar Guidelines

The Guidelines have been implemented in various practice settings, which indicates they are transferable outside the settings in where they were developed and was one evaluation site
• They became policy at Barwon Health in 2014, which indicates they are sustainable after the research was completed
• Medical record audits undertaken before the Guidelines were implemented in 2014 and approximately nine months after implementation show changes consistent with the Guidelines in McKellar Centre residents' care plans including evidence that care is personalised, e.g. blood glucose monitoring and care plan is based on the person's hypoglycaemia risk
• Barwon Health staff is required to attend annual professional development sessions that encompass The McKellar guidelines
• The risk assessment tools were translated into Norwegian and being used in Norway in research and practice
• The Guidelines were cited in the Australian Government Australian National Diabetes Strategy 2016–2020
• They are a component of Module 7 of an online self-directed learning programme offered by the Australian National Association of Diabetes Centres (NADC)
• The Guidelines led to several peer-review and invited papers and presentations including presenting at the National Better Practice Conferences, the NADC Best Practice Conference and Sigma Theta Tau International Conference
• They were awarded the Barwon Healthcare Innovation Award in 2013 and the Barwon Health Quality Award in 2016 and were a finalist in the Victorian Quality Awards in 2016

examples of how HPs can use the information to plan care with older people with diabetes.

Implementing any new initiative can be challenging, especially when the local context/situation is not considered. The Knowledge-to-Action framework helped HPs decide the facilitators and barriers and context-specific issues in their practice settings. Considering the specific care context enabled HPs to decide which care topic and risk assessment tools were relevant to their particular care setting. HPs should decide which Guidelines and Risk Assessment Tools are most relevant to their population of older people with diabetes and the advantages, benefits and risks of implementing The Guidelines, agree on an implementation process and implementation team and the roles and responsibilities of the implementation team. The Guidelines must be easily accessible in practice settings.

4.10   Using The McKellar Guidelines to Personalise Care

HPs can use one or all of the five RATs to determine key risks for each individual older person and then develop strategies with them to manage their risks. Risk assessment can be undertaken during any consultation and can also occur as part of the Annual Cycle of Care (ACC) and during the *Health Assessment for People Aged 75 and Old*er (Dunning et al. 2013a; Dunning 2016), when health status changes, after admission to an RACF and after a hospital admission. Older people are at increased risk of readmission within 30 days especially for medicine-related errors and adverse events (Caughey et al. 2017).

HPs can use The Guidelines to plan care for older people with diabetes living in an RACF. Our medical record audits in RACFs identified three particular issues that need to be addressed:

- Undertaking risk assessment for undiagnosed diabetes when an older person is admitted to an RACF. We found ~50% of older people in RACF with no diagnosis of diabetes were at risk using the AUSD risk tool.
- Using reportable blood glucose ranges, many of which are unsafe.
- Using stat (top up) doses of insulin to treat isolated episodes of hyperglycaemia. Top up doses lead to hypoglycaemia and rebound hyperglycaemia and associated adverse events such as falls (Cheung and Chipps 2010; American Geriatrics Society 2015). These adverse consequences associated with stat insulin doses were documented in the 1960s (Cheung and Chipps 2010; American Geriatrics Society 2015). Continued use reflects outdated practice.

4.11   Continuing Medical Education

The Guidelines and *The McKellar Way* can also be used as the basis for diabetes-related continuing professional development programmes in individual practices and workshops at conferences. Such CME activities could encompass how to implement them in routine primary care.

4.12   Summary

This chapter highlighted key issues concerning guidelines, decision aids and shared decision-making. It used The McKellar Guidelines as an example of a process that might enhance knowledge translation and uptake of other guidelines in the future.

4.13   Reflection Point

- Think about decision-making and how your values, experiences, attitudes and knowledge could influence the way you engage with older people with diabetes.

References

American Geriatrics Society (2015) Beers Criteria Update Expert Panel (2015) American Geriatrics Society 2015 updated beers criteria for potentially inappropriate medication use in older adults. J Am Geriatr Soc 63(11):2227–2246

Bayer Tadd (2006)

Carmen K, Dardess P, Maurer M et al (2013) Patient and family engagement: a framework for understanding the elements and developing interventions and policies. Health Aff 32(2):223–231

Caughey G, Pratt N, Barratt J et al (2017) Understanding 30 day re-admission after hospitalisation of older patients for diabetes: identifying those at greatest risk. Med J Aust 208(4):170–175

Chapman S (2017) What matters most to you? How decision aids help patients make better choices. http://www.evidentlycochrane.net/what-matters-most-to-youe-how-decision-aids-help-patients-make-beter-choices-2/

Cheung Chips (2010)

Corriere M, Minang L, Sisson S et al (2014) The use of clinical guidelines highlights ongoing educational gaps in physician's knowledge and decision making related to diabetes. BMC Med Educ. https://doi.org/10.1186/1472-6920-14-186

Da Vinci L (1452–1519) Knowing is not enough. https://www.goodreads.com/.../146988-i-have-been-impressed-with-the-urgency-of-doing-knowing

Dunning T (2016) Assessing older people with diabetes in Australia. Prim Care Diabetes Soc Aust 1(4):115–120

Dunning T, Savage S, Duggan N (2013a) A philosophical framework to guide care of older people with diabetes. Centre for Nursing and Allied Health Research and IDOP, Melbourne

Dunning T, Savage S, Duggan N (2013b) The McKellar guidelines for managing older people with diabetes in residential and other care settings. Deakin University and Barwon Health, Geelong Centre for Nursing and Allied Health Research

Field B, Booth A, Ilott I, Gerrish K (2014) Using the knowledge to action framework in practice: a citation analysis and systematic review. Implement Sci 9:172. https://doi.org/10.1186/s13012-014-0172-2. PMCID: PMC4258036

Glasgow R, Emmons K (2007) How can we increase translation of research into practice. Types of evidence needed. Annu Rev Public Health 28:413–433

Graham ID, Logan J, Harrison MB, Straus SE, Tetroe J, Caswell W, Robinson N. Lost in knowledge translation: time for a map? J Contin Educ Heal Prof 2006;26(1):13–24

Graham I, Logrin J, Harrison MB et al (2006) Lost in translation: time for a roadmap? J Contin Educ Health Prof 26(1):13–20

Green W, Ottoson J, Garcia C, Hiatt R (2009) Diffusion theory and knowledge dissemination, utilisation and integration in public health. Annu Rev Public Health 30:151–174

Grenhalghh T, MacFarlane R, Bate F et al (2004) Diffusion of innovations in service organisations: systematic review and recommendations. Millbank Q 82(4):581–629

Harris J, Graue M, Dunning T et al (2015) Involving people with diabetes and the wider community in diabetes research: a realist review protocol. Syst Rev. https://doi.org/10.1185/s13643-015-0127-y

International Diabetes Federation (IDF) (2013) Global guideline for managing older people with type 2 diabetes. www.idf.org. Accessed July 2017

Kadu M, Stolee P (2015) Facilitators and barriers to implementing the chronic disease model in primary care: a systematic review. BMC Fam Pract. https://doi.org/10.1186/s12875-014-0219-0

Malterud (2001)

Modern English–Old English dictionary. www.majstro.com/dictionaries/English-Old%20English/heal. Accessed October 2017

National Health and Medical Research Council (1995) Guideline for the development and implementation of clinical practice guidelines. Australian Publishing Service, Canberra

Nugent Pam. Psychological distance in *PsychologyDictionary.org*, April 28, 2013. https://psychologydictionary.org/psychological-distance/ Accessed 30 Oct 2017

Stacey D, Higuchi KA, Menard P, Davies B, Graham ID, O'Connor AM. Integrating patient decision support in an undergraduate nursing curriculum: an implementation project. Int J Nurs Educ Scholarsh 2009;6:10. https://doi.org/10.2202/1548-923X.1741

Starfield B (2011) Is patient-centred care the same as person-focused care? Permanete J 15(2):63–69

Trope Y, Liberman N (2010) Construal-level theory of psychological distance. Psychol Rev 117(2):440

Turner T, Misso M, Harris C, Green S (2008) Development of evidence-based clinical practice guidelines (CPGs): comparing approaches. Implement Sci. https://doi.org/10.1186/1748-5008-3-45

Weiner S (2004) From research to evidence to context: the challenge of individualizing care. Ann Intern Med 141(3):141–145

World Health Organisation (WHO) (2017) WHO handbook of guideline development, 2nd edn. WHO, Geneva. http://www.who.int/publications/guideline/handbook_2nd_ed.pdf. Accessed Oct 2017

WHO (2017b) Integrated care for older people. WHO, Geneva. www.who.int/ageing. Accessed Oct 2017

WHO (2017c) WHO definition of palliative care. http://www.who.int/cancer/palliative/definition/en/. Accessed July 2017

Nutrition and Exercise: A Personalised Approach

5

Sital Harris

Let food by thy medicine and medicine be thy food (Hippocrates 460–375 BCE)

Key Points

- The use of clinical tools to assess nutritional status has a valid role to make decisions about the individual nutritional needs and early nutritional intervention.
- Exercise for older people is an essential therapy for mental and physical well-being.
- A holistic approach to personal nutrition considers faith, personal wishes, ethical view of the individual, personal food behaviours and preferences.
- The art to personal nutrition involves regular meal planning and targeting specific nutrients based on individual needs.
- Personal exercise and nutritional plans contribute to good glycaemic control and healthy ageing.

5.1 A Nutritional Therapists Approach to Personal Nutritional and Physical Activity Care: A Review of the Evidence

The term 'healthy diet' is frequently used to describe a diet that is balanced in nutrition. Ideally each meal will be balanced with a source of protein, carbohydrates, fruits or vegetables, fibre and low in saturated fats, salt and sugar. Healthy snacks

S. Harris, M.Sc., R.N.T.
Foundation for Diabetes Research in Older People, Luton, UK
e-mail: sital@responsiva.biz

© Springer International Publishing AG, part of Springer Nature 2018
T. Dunning (ed.), *The Art and Science of Personalising Care with Older People with Diabetes*, https://doi.org/10.1007/978-3-319-74360-8_5

can be consumed in between meals to help with blood glucose control. An example of such a meal might be grilled chicken, steamed mixed garden vegetables, new potatoes and a light olive oil, parsley and vinegar dressing, a piece of fruit with a pot of yogurt and oatmeal crackers with a piece of cheese or some nut butter. A healthy diet provides us with the nutrients to stay fit, healthy and providing us with energy, whilst nourishing our body with quality nutrients to keep us fit and healthy. Each part of a meal should have a function and nutritional purpose to keep our body and mind fit, healthy and to fight off illness or infections. For an older person, illness can be a physical illness or a mental illness such as depression.

Calorie needs do change with age because our basal metabolic rate (BMR) slows down; this is because older people are less active. Our BMR is the rate at which we expend energy whilst at rest. Factors likely to change someone's BMR include less physical activity, emotional stress, depression and illness or infection. Sadly, many older people are likely to experience stress, depression, illness and infections; therefore, the quality of their diet perhaps has more meaning to keeping them well and reduce the risk of frailty. Diet therapy plays even a bigger part if they have diabetes, which requires self-monitoring and glycaemic control through diet and exercise.

It is assumed that because older people are less active, they may not need as many calories or that they can 'eat what they like because they are older' or 'they are old, let them enjoy their food'. Whilst there is some truth in these views, we should recognise that older people still do require a balanced healthy diet to keep them well and prevent frailty. Personal nutrition allows for each meal to be tailored to meet the individual nutritional needs. It is reasonable to perhaps increase some nutrients such as protein or fibre when the individual is feeling unwell or suffering from stress. Evidence is now emerging to suggest we should take a longer-term strategy to develop better personal dietary interventions for older people, the reason being to prevent frailty (McClure and Villani 2017).

5.2   The Role of a Healthy Diet

A healthy balanced diet and regular activity are essential components to health and well-being (Ngandu et al. 2015). Using personal nutrition and exercise can protect an older person from sarcopenia and the onset of frailty (Robinson et al. 2016). Personalising nutritional care considers the many personalities and behaviours of older people as these are likely to influence their food preferences more so (Iwasa et al. 2008). Personalities and behaviours can change if older people are in pain or emotionally upset.

An older person's diet needs to be balanced and they need regular physical activity to prevent frailty (Dominguez and Barbagallo 2017). Both support older people emotionally which is equally important to healthy ageing. Behaviour change and age have no barriers—older people can and are willing to make dietary changes to improve their health and well-being (Beverly et al. 2013); health professionals should include the older person in decisions about dietary needs and changes to help improve overall diabetes and well-being (Heisler et al. 2007). The emphasis is on effective communication by the clinicians or carers to take time to work with older people to personalise the nutritional needs and diabetes management. One should remember older people are not difficult to work with because of their habits or behaviours; they merely need time, compassion and respect, especially when discussing the need to adhere to a healthy diet. Older people may need time to adjust to new dietary changes or advice however, they are willing to learn and change if given the support and encouragement. Older people can have complex medical conditions aside from their diabetes; this would influence their approach to dietary interventions. Dialogue is therefore quite an important skill to learn and develop when personalising nutritional care.

Personal nutrition is about using a holistic approach that offers appropriate nutrition for the individual needs and even at specific times. It is about discussion and engagement with the individual, so when they suggest they are too old to change, I would politely suggest they are able to improve diet and enjoy the entire process of personal nutrition. I am likely to encourage them to tell me a 'story' about their favourite meal or a special event; this technique helps to engage in conversation and I can make small suggestions or changes and allow for us to compromise—thus the beginning of a healthy and happy working relationship between myself and the individual.

We become a team with a joint aim to improve their nutritional status. The scenario might go as 'so George, I bet you can tell me some wonderful stories about your favourite foods when you were a young lad'. George sings like a canary to tell me all about his worst and favourite meals, he also begins to open about his current meals, what he likes and what he does not like. We talk about his COPD and how this affects his enjoyment of food. I can now suggest some changes and we agree these together. This conversation outlines the route to George's challenge and frustrations with meal times, something I might not have fully understood if I had not entered a relaxed conversation about food with George. This is my take on helping older individuals with behaviour change and dietary changes to improve their nutrition and help achieve better health outcomes (García-Esquinas et al. 2015). Health professionals need to consider time as an important factor for personalising nutritional needs for older people, especially if they have diabetes.

Such a discussion allows me to consider the actual food, how it is farmed, absorbed, digested, cellular function, metabolising, excretion, their medical conditions, physiological requirements, possible nutrient and drug interactions, and emotional well-being. Could they be under- and overconsumption of some foods, alcohol misuse, and safety of foods specifically for everyone. Nutrient quality is perhaps more important than calorie counting, at least in the initial stages of supporting and changing dietary habits in older people (Ley et al. 2014). It may be better for the individual to have smaller meals but they are nutrient dense. An example of this may be scrambled eggs with a slice of toast.

The link between personalising nutritional support, achieving stable diabetes control and thus preventing frailty and premature death in older people with diabetes is strong enough to give rationale to personating nutritional care for older people, and move away from the views or behaviour that older people cannot or will not change their diet to improve their health and well-being (Castro-Rodríguez et al. 2016). The aim is to keep older people fit and healthy so there is a decent quality of life in later years.

Stable blood glucose levels are a key to achieving stable diabetes control; factors that help influence this are eating attitudes and behaviours to adhering to a healthy diet, and a healthy BMI; diet therapy can contribute to good glycaemic control. I would further consider their emotional well-being as part of my personal nutrition.

Individuals with diabetes have a higher risk of developing physical disabilities; this risk increases further with age (Bianchi et al. 2013). Our ageing population is growing and more older individuals are at risk of geriatric syndromes such as dementia and falls (Corriere et al. 2013). It is reasonable that even frailty may accelerate Alzheimer disease and age-related cognitive function, possibly more so in frailer women than in frailer men (Kojima et al. 2016).

Dementia and frailty have a strong link and it is understandable that older individuals may reduce their physical activities and nutritional status because of such decline in both physical and mental health (Kojima et al. 2016). Often, they can experience a loss of appetite or they struggle to prepare foods physically, simple tasks like opening a jar or draining a hot pan with cooked pasta might become a challenge. Simple tasks in the kitchen can even cause injury such as small burns or joint pain if they lift sometimes too heavy. Those living alone may be mindful of the costs of cooking or a healthy hot meal. Sometimes they may have experienced an incident in the kitchen, which could have caused injury or frustration; such an experience could prevent them from cooking meals. It therefore seems an easier option to snack on cakes, biscuits or convenience foods.

Cognitive function may be associated with nutrient deficiency in iron and B12, both common in older people (Andro et al. 2013). Older adults may have difficulty in B12 absorption despite sufficient amounts consumed through diet or through supplementation (Paul and Selub 2017). A B12 deficiency can further compromise cognitive function if the current diet is sufficient in folate but not sufficient in B12 (Moore et al. 2014).

Older people are at risk of iron deficiency, often compromised because of chronic health conditions like kidney disease and heart conditions (Lopez et al. 2016). Kidney disease and cardiovascular conditions are common in those with diabetes and adding another layer of risk for frailer individuals with diabetes. Low levels of iron may contribute to cognitive decline in older individuals (Andro et al. 2013). A decline may even begin with mild forms of depression or even loneliness.

The evidence suggests that nutrition is a very relevant component to preventing frailty and cognitive decline in our older population (Dominguez and Barbagallo 2017). The link between the nutritional status and how frailty develops is strong, even suggesting that some nutrients are more important to prevent frailty such as proteins and vitamin D. Frailty may develop at a faster pace when the individual is lacking in nutrients, therefore telling us how important diet and nutrition is for older people in general (Artaza-Artabe et al. 2016). We can understand frailty syndrome and malnutrition using tools like the mini nutritional assessment (MNA) to identify frailty early or at 'risk of frailty' to then support individuals with personal nutritional care because malnutrition can lead to older people becoming weaker and frail (Bollwein et al. 2013).

The MNA tool has been used as a reliable assessment tool to predict the nutritional status of older people; it considers BMI, low muscle mass, reduction in mobility, and all common signs of early stage frailty (Kan and Vellas 2011). The nutritional can help identify the individual's nutritional status e.g. whether they are well nourished, undernourished or malnourished the older individual is according to a score that helps to guide nutritional interventions (Schrader et al. 2014). Poor nutrition often develops due to a lack of calories and appropriate hydration in older people, both likely to contribute to severe weight loss in older people.

Weight loss is another contributory factor for developing frailty amongst older individuals. Unfortunately, significant weight loss is a characteristic of anorexia nervosa and likely to occur in older individuals who simply find it hard to eat. In these individuals severe weight loss occurs and muscle strength and appetite decline. For some older and frailer individuals weight loss is a common health concern; once severe weight loss begins, it can be harder to support individuals to regain appetite and weight (Morley 2012). This is why early nutritional intervention can delay or prevent frailty syndrome.

Older people who have diabetes are at further risk of lower levels of strength in leg muscle (Park et al. 2007), a reduction in gait speed and grip strength likely to be because of a combination of diabetes and sarcopenia. These factors will affect their ability to walk or take part in physical activity (Volpato et al. 2012). It may influence their own desire to try and build muscle strength or take part in any form of physical activity. Raised blood glucose levels are likely to contribute to increased risk of disabilities which can also lead to frailty (Lu et al. 2009). Hyperglycaemia seems to be a reliable early predictor to preliminary stages of frailty (Kalyani et al. 2015).

A plausible reason may be that they eat a diet high in convenience foods to provide them with energy, examples include biscuits, sugar in hot drinks and cakes. These types of food provide energy and they are easily accessible but they are not necessarily nutritionally appropriate. The need to intervene with appropriate nutritional therapy is necessary to help slow the speed of frailty and for individuals who are pre-frail. The evidence suggests a clear link with diabetes, sarcopenia, frailty and malnutrition.

5.3 How to Select Healthier and Appropriate Foods

The ageing process naturally slows down protein metabolism and synthesis (Kumar et al. 2009) suggesting that additional protein would be necessary to reduce muscle loss in older people. The optimal protein should be personal especially for those with chronic conditions like kidney disease but protein still needs to form a significant component to nutritional intervention and advice. Approximately a third of the total daily calories should come from protein sources, for some individual this may need a slight increase or decrease depending on other health conditions (Bauer et al. 2013).

Specific amino acid like leucine which is rich in whey proteins help improve protein synthesis and aid recovery following exercise and from illness. It is therefore beneficial for older people to develop muscle growth and strength through appropriate protein intake (Burd et al. 2012). Leucine is one of the eight essential amino acids needed for protein synthesis and development of muscle mass; food sources include legumes, beef and fish.

Eating 2 pieces of oily fish provides essential fatty acids and is a reliable source of quality protein. Oily fish may prevent retinopathy in older individuals with diabetes, so this protein source has many nutritional benefits (Sala-Vila et al. 2016). Fish is generally a lighter meat to digest. Older adults do have challenges with nutrient absorption because the intestine walls lose elasticity through the ageing process and older people tend to have lower levels of hydrochloric acid, resulting in additional bacterial growth in the gut walls. Some older individuals are likely to experience discomfort or pain when eating large or specific meals. Therefore, diet choice needs careful planning and personalising to suit the individual health needs, whilst minimising digestive discomfort.

Oily fish is a key component to the Mediterranean diet and this diet is a favourable diet for older people to follow because this diet is based on legumes, fresh fruits, vegetables and oily fish (Artaza-Artabe et al. 2016). Whilst the Mediterranean diet has been well researched, the essence of this diet is fresh foods so the concept of this diet does suit many cultures and culinary tastes from Eastern flavours to South-Asian cuisine dishes. The concept is adaptable. Oily fish is a rich source of the sunshine vitamin D, which is necessary for calcium absorption and muscle development and muscle function. Vitamin D contributes to a stronger skeletal strength and muscle mass (Beaudart et al. 2014). Unfortunately, many older people do suffer with vitamin D deficiency.

The Mediterranean style diet is likely to improve memory and cognitive function in older people when combined with physical activity and memory training to slow down cognitive decline and keep individuals healthy physically and mentally throughout the ageing process (Ngandu et al. 2015). The Mediterranean diet is naturally rich in fibre, vitamins, minerals, healthy oils and proteins; it is a natural diet using whole and unprocessed foods. There is scope for versatility to suit many tastes and textures when developing menus and meal plans with this diet. The other component to this diet is the 'lifestyle' factor suggesting a relaxed approach to meal planning and mealtimes does contribute to older people eating a better diet and enjoying healthier foods.

5.4   The Role of Supplementation and Feeds

For some frail individuals chewing and eating foods may not be an option due to a poor health; therefore, oral nutritional supplementation (ONS) and even enteral feeds may be necessary to support the individual for their nutritional needs. One still needs to consider a personal approach through discussion with the individual where possible, family members and the clinical staff so an appropriate and safe choice is made for the health and well-being of the individual. Factors such as faith are a critical consideration when using enteral feeds (Greenberger 2015), one needs to remember everyone still requires a personal approach when the need arises for medical intervention with feeds and ONS. Enteral feeds do have a place to support individuals at risk of malnutrition or already malnourished individuals but they come with ethical challenges and one needs to consider faith, beliefs, infections and practical use of such interventions for older people.

There is considerable risk of infections and further complications when using ONS or enteral feeds and careful and ethical consideration needs to form a key component to making the choice to use these (Cintra et al. 2014). These considerations are even more important for older individuals with advanced stage of dementia and dysphagia, so the question of quality of life and dignity need to be discussed openly with individuals when possible, family and the wider clinical team (Goldberg and Altman 2014). Making the decision to use a feed is a difficult one because one needs to think carefully about the individual's personal needs and wishes, perhaps even more than the actual clinical decision. Feeds are complex nutritional solutions that can be used in a clinical setting; personal care may not be a factor in the decision-making process to use a feed, maybe because they are a medical intervention. The use of feeds can still be personalised to consider the flavours of ONS or time of an enteral feed.

5.5 The Evidence for Exercise and Frailty

Exercise for older people with diabetes has been shown to improve frailty and improve health and well-being in older people (Beaudart et al. 2014). The aim of regular exercise is to strengthen muscles which give the individual structure, movement and for many this physical change can improve mood and self-confidence. Strength in muscles can prevent frailty and falls in older people and it can take away fear of falling. More specifically, weight-bearing exercises work well to build muscle mass and gain strength. Stretching and gentle walking help to build confidence and increase movement. Socially exercise helps to stimulate the brain and release happy hormones.

Many older people may fear a fall or muscle weakness; this becomes a psychological barrier to doing exercise and trying to improve muscle strength. Therefore, it is important to start slowly and use exercise to improve grip strength, coordination and confidence. The reason for early physical intervention is to prevent frailty in the first instance but further to support those with some elements of frailty and help reduce further weakness in the muscle. Strength-bearing and weight-bearing exercises appear to be the most relevant methods for healthy ageing (Serra-Prat et al. 2017).

For some individuals, strength-bearing exercises may not be suitable in the initial assessments, alternatives methods include gentle walking to then build up speed and balance testing to appropriate limitations (Heiland et al. 2016). Physical activity contributes to mental well-being and even alertness in those with dementia (Telenius et al. 2015), suggesting all older individuals are capable of some form of physical activity, some may require support or assistance but all need to be encouraged to get active and be involved with lifestyle, physical activity and nutritional interventions for healthy ageing. I would suggest small steps to then build up over a few weeks or months. Part of this is to build confidence and muscle mass.

5.6 How to Achieve Small but Significant Nutritional and Physical Activity Changes to Improve Diabetes Control and Reduce Frailty: My Personal Approach

When considering personal nutrition, the key is to keep changing the formula to suit the individual nutritional needs at that specific time or period, this involves personal meal planning frequently at each meal. I may not necessarily base my meal plans on a person's size, shape or weight but I am likely to base my planning on their energy and food preferences in the initial stages. It can help to gather a food and drink dairy prior to any assessment to help appreciate current eating patterns. You have to have a starting point to move forward and improve nutritional intake. The aim is to improve nutritional status and not necessary calories alone.

5.7   How and When to Use Clinical Data

Using clinical data like blood results, MNA and health records guide me to selecting specific foods that are nutrient dense rather than calorie dense. When managing people with diabetes, one should consider stable blood glucose levels so 'little and often' and 'nutrient dense' are two methods that help achieve glycaemic control and increase necessary nutrients like proteins, iron and B12 in the diet. Allergies and drug nutrient interactions need to be identified before planning meals. Many older people can suffer from food intolerances, and these are not the same as food allergies; intolerances simply suggest the individual may suffer from digestive discomfort when eating some foods.

5.8   How to Personalise Enteral Feeding

When the need arises to use ONS or enteral feeds, one needs to select these carefully and tailor the feed to the individual and their diabetes. Factors to consider are allergy feeds, gluten free, controlled protein for some health conditions, dairy free, glucose levels and flavours of the feeds. Personal nutrition in such cases requires that health workers check that the individual is happy and comfortable with the feed. Appropriate insulin during the feed is critical, especially in those with type 1 diabetes. Regular blood glucose testing before and after feeds is important. The length of time of feed needs to be discussed because some may prefer the feed over night or throughout the day. Enteral feeds should be checked regularly to ensure they have not become blocked or stopped. The risk of infection increases with feeds and healthcare professionals should take time with the individual to ensure their feed is safe, secure and comfortable.

Personal nutrition in this case considers the individual wishes of when they want their feeds, and one needs to respect any restrictions on using feeds based on personal or ethical beliefs. Faith is a huge part of many of us and respect for each faith is critical when considering enteral feeding (Greenberger 2015). Every aspect of enteral feeding or ONS need to be carefully explained where possible. In situations where the individual becomes upset, it may be wise to allow the individual time and listen to any concerns or fears. ONS can be high in sugars, they come in a variety of flavours, some flavours are acceptable for individuals and some may not be, personal preferences are important to ensure individual compliance. If the feed is unpalatable, then the individual is unlikely to finish the feed and at risk of malnutrition. Appropriate insulin or diabetic medication needs to be administered in a timely manner. Delays in medication and feeds can cause hypoglycaemia or hyperglycaemia.

5.9   How to Personalise Meals

Personalising nutritional needs for older people with diabetes is about considering recipes at the heart of personal care. Once I understand the individual's values, needs, wishes and food relationships, I can create meal plans which are nutritious and personal so they have meaning and purpose for the individual. Meals become enjoyable again and adding a richness for older people. Personal meal plans offer the individual to remember special times and meals because they bring back memories, emotions and stories, whilst still considering the medical and nutritional needs for the individual. The aim is to ensure regular meals that are rich in protein, fruits and vegetables, so little and often the key to my success.

I begin this process by asking about their daily routines, social clubs, foods they enjoy and why. Dialogue helps to engage with older people generally and dialogue helps to communicate the importance of good nutritional care, physical activity to well-being and healthy ageing. Having one specific group of foods is likely to result in some form of malnourishment. Many older people can have limited variety because of health issues, mobility, unable to cook or even cost of preparing meals. This is where dialogue helps to uncover such issues to help overcome some issues whilst being mindful of others. If my patients really did not like eating fruits then I simply would not recommend these or even discuss these, instead, perhaps looking at increasing vegetables or proteins that are equally nutritionally appropriate. There is no hard and fast rule to eat every food group or food type.

Our diet needs to comprise of seven food groups: carbohydrates, fruits and vegetables, proteins, dairy or dairy alternatives and healthy fats. Nutrients from our foods (diet); therefore, we don't superficially eat nutrients but food. Recipes create meals—this is the link between nutrition, food and personal diabetes care. Recipes which have been shared amongst friends, family, through cooking methods, cooking facilities, festivities, faith, through communities, generations and cultures, this is really where our nutrition comes from—people. This connection and understanding helps to create a personal approach. It is about asking questions and learning from what the individual tells you about their relationship with food, cooking and nutrition. I have created meal plans based on war-time recipes and methods to help encourage an older person to increase their calories and protein, these menus have since created joyful discussions and engagement to help increase nutrients and food intake. This principle can apply to a care home setting. The key is to prepare meals using fresh foods when possible and minimise processed foods.

It is good to involve family or the care setting because often they are likely preparing meals. Based on these discussions, the aim needs to be to have regular but smaller meals that have a quality source of protein, plenty of fruits and some vegetables. Calcium and vitamin D contribute to muscle development and healthy bones. Smaller meals but often may be the better option to increase nutritional status of older people. A healthy nutritious diet and strength-bearing exercises help to prevent sarcopenia and the onset of frailly; it is this combined approach that seems to support individuals develop muscle strength and improve muscle function (Deutz et al. 2014).

It is reasonable for health professionals to prescribe a course of planned personal meals and exercise routines that are personal to individual needs and improve physical strength. This method is likely to improve overall health and well-being—thus reduce risk of frailty (de Souto Barreto et al. 2016). Such programmes can be tailored using modern technology for those who are home-bound or in a care home setting, using technology ensures older people are still involved and able to take part in physical and mental exercises (Hong et al. 2017). I often use personal prescriptions which outline key nutrients and exercises to support an older person with diabetes and who may be at risk of frailty. This prescription supports them to make changes to achieve stable diabetes, maintain strength and improve nutritional status. Malnutrition in older people is common; small changes and early intervention can prevent malnutrition from developing.

5.10   The Role of Hydration

Hydration is a critical factor to survival, unfortunately for older people, keeping hydrated might not seem a priority to health and well-being. Physical strength and disabilities might be a reason; however, specialist cups and support need to be discussed with everyone to ensure that in the initial instance they are physically able to drink (Campbell 2016). Poor hydration is likely to lead to inferior quality of life and poor outcomes for individuals who have been hospitalised (El-Sharkawy et al. 2015). All foods and drink contain fluids; if drinking is a challenge then my strategy would be to encourage fruits and water-based vegetables. I may encourage extra pieces of water-based fruits to snack on, watermelon, grapes, pears, strawberries. I might offer a fresh glass of water or diluted squash in between meals and I am likely to encourage them to drink it.

I may consider small sticks of peeled cucumber with a cheese dip. I may even use fruit and vegetable smoothies as a mid-morning or mid-afternoon snack. Again, my method is small cups, small volumes but frequently. I may not encourage a jug of water on the side, as this limits their movement where possible and often this water is not fresh. It's perhaps good to encourage them to get up and get a fresh glass of water, tea or fruit quash. For those who are unable to walk, caregivers need to offer fluids regularly and allow them time to finish a small drink. It is important to consider potential cognitive decline and accelerated risk of frailty for those in a hospital or care home setting (McCrow et al. 2016).

Unfortunately, when dehydration occurs, the likelihood of quality of life and nutritional status may be affected. Dehydration can compromise compliance and individuals can seem to be difficult when in truth, this change in behaviour is likely due to dehydration. The view to consider is any form of fluids is better than no or limited fluids. Consider all forms of hydration from tea, diluted fruit juice, fruit cordials, boiled water with a slice of lemon, tap water, fruit or herbal teas. Tiny amounts of fluid may be more manageable. Sometimes they may need company whilst having a drink, this can encourage them to finish a drink.

Key Considerations
- The art to considering personal nutritional needs is to understand what the individual wishes are, then consider the individual nutritional needs to plan meals. This may involve a different approach to dialogue, improved listening skills and

teamwork between the individual, carers and my nutritional recommendations. Listening skills help to understand underlying issues which can prevent the individual from adhering to a healthy diet. Allow the individual to tell you stories because this aspect helps to understand the individual's relationships with food. Make minor changes regularly because nutritional needs will change frequently. I use a variety of recipe books to tailor meals and inspire and re-engage individuals with food. For me, meal planning is the key element to ensure an older person with diabetes has a balanced diet that supports them to stay fit and healthy. I consult regularly with health professionals and individuals to develop individual nutrition plans. Meal planning for older people is a skill I have developed over many years and through experience of working with older people living with diabetes.

- Adequate protein, vitamin D, fruits and vegetables and regular exercise work well together. This combination helps to strengthen muscles and helps to prevent frailty. I would consider the quality of protein instead of the quantity. It is my preference they eat smaller amounts of quality proteins throughout the day or week over eating larger meals. I believe in smaller meals but on a frequent basis. This helps to ensure the individual is nourished and hydrated. It is reasonable to use smoothies and soups to help increase proteins, fluids and nutrition. Consider a mix of animal- and plant-based proteins to increase protein diversity. There are now wonderful plant-based proteins which are easier to digest for older people and they may be a better alternative to help increase protein intake.
- A personal prescription of exercise and nutrition play a significant role in preventing frailty and reduces the risk of sarcopenia. It is important to outline this link when possible, so they appreciate why their diet and exercise is important.
- Ensure the individual is hydrated with regular fresh fluids—consider personal preferences with each drink. Dehydration can lead to confusion, depression, constipation and discomfort. Soft fruits are a reliable source of fibre and fluids, and smoothies and lollipops are good snack options.
- I would consider gut health because older people can suffer from bloating, acid reflux, abdominal cramps and pain; these can limit their choice of foods and quantity. Using a probiotic or a live-yogurt drink is worth discussing with the individual and their family. Gut discomfort is a common reason why an older person may have limited dietary intake; understanding this can help support them to find foods they can tolerate.

When I am developing a meal plan or offering nutritional advice/guidance, I am mindful that once the individual leaves my consultation, they become a consumer. Consumers are targeted with marketing messages on food packaging, supermarket offers and 'special savings'—messages that may influence the choices they make when purchasing food. My influence and advice can be diluted by such marketing messages. Therefore, I factor such marketing and health claims when offering advice. I may even discuss which supermarket they shop at or offer advice on specific brands or types of food.

Fig. 5.1 Framework for personalising nutrition information

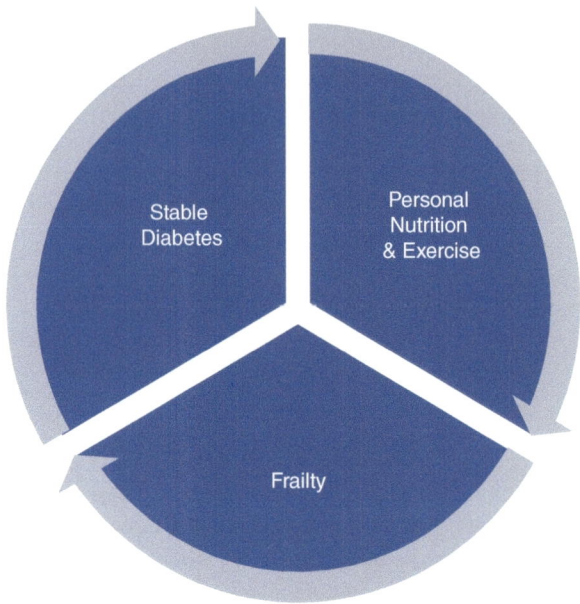

I often use recipes and prepare a shopping list of things to consider when purchasing food; these are personal and specific to each individual nutritional need; my recipes do change with each visit to encourage new foods and home cooking. Cost is another factor I think about when offering individual care because cost is most likely to influence the individual more if they are on a low budget. I use seasonal products because this can help keep costs low. I may outline the meaning of health claims on food packaging or explain terms like 'low-fat' or 'fat-free', these are terms used on food packaging to influence consumer spend. It is simpler to offer recipes that encompass the correct nutrients as a starting point. This works well with older people because they use this list/recipe to buy the foods suitable for their needs. Below is a small selection of recipes I may use to encourage healthy eating; these recipes are simple and nutritious.

My interpretation of personal nutrition is to work with the individual and their family/carer to develop suitable meals that are enjoyable, cost effective and nutritious. Nutrition should also encompass quality of life—meals need to be enjoyable.

The following three figures are the author's frameworks designed to be used during consultations and when personalising nutritional care (Figs. 5.1, 5.2, and 5.3).

5.11   Recipes for Hydration

Constipation and dehydration are common in older people, smoothies help to hydrate because many fruits and vegetables are water based, they provide fibre, vitamins and minerals. Most importantly, they can be sweet and easy to digest.

Fig. 5.2 Sample Meal Plan Structures to personalise meal plans

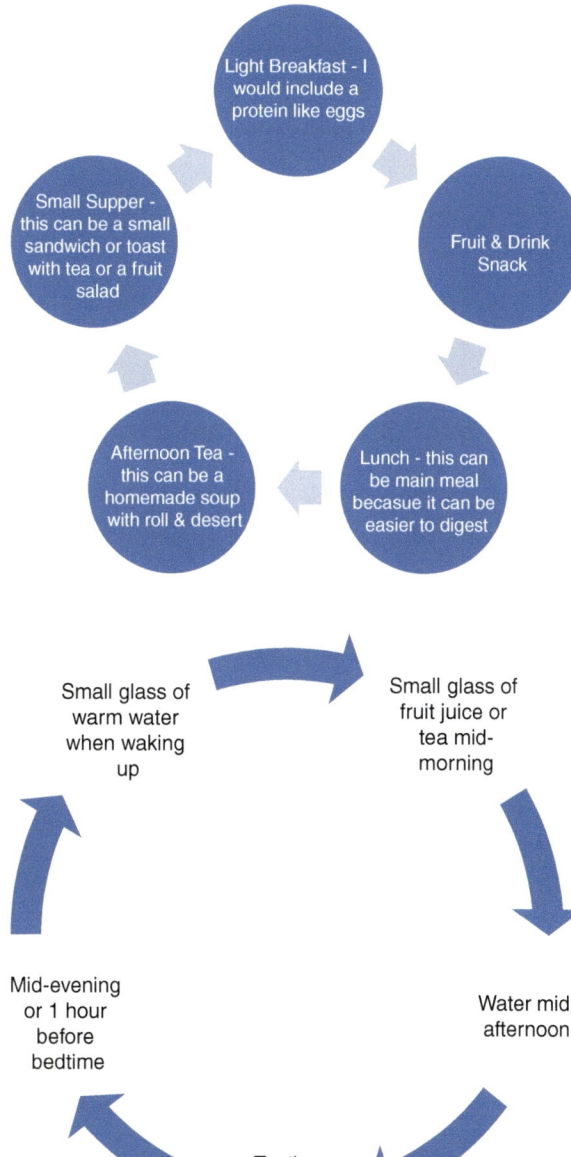

Fig. 5.3 Sample plan to maintain hydration

Energy Boost Smoothie—Makes 4–5 portions

300 g Tofu, 2 ripe bananas, half a fresh mango, small cup of soya milk, 1tbsp honey.

Roughly chop the fruits and tofu and place in a blender. Add the honey and milk, then blend the ingredients together. Add additional milk to adjust consistency if necessary. Serve in small glass. You can use apple juice or a different milk if preferred. This smoothie is rich in protein, vitamins C, B and potassium. It is an excellent choice for a mid-morning snack or even a lighter breakfast option. You can add a little ground cinnamon and cardamom to spice it up.

Pear and Peaches Delight—Makes two portions

2 Ripe pears, 2 ripe peaches (remove skins if necessary), small banana, small cup of apple juice and a pinch of cinnamon (optional).

Roughly chop the fruits and place in a blender. Add the juice and cinnamon if using. Blend the ingredients together, ensure all the consistency is OK and serve with some crushed ice. This drink is a reliable source of vitamins B, C, fibre and potassium. Remove the banana for those you need a low potassium diet.

Berries, Berries and Berries—Makes three small portions

Use a handful of blueberries, blackberries, strawberries and raspberries. 150 natural or fruit yogurt, 1 tbsp. of honey, small amount of milk.

Place all the ingredients into a blender and blend well until the fruits are broken down. Add additional milk if required to adjust the consistency for the individual. This smoothie is a reliable source of vitamin C, calcium, B2, B6 and folic acid.

5.12   Recipes for Protein

Protein helps to build muscle mass, using a combination of animal- and plant-based proteins provides variety. Plant-based proteins like legumes and peas may be easier to digest for some. White meats are softer and a lighter meat option. Consider offal because of the high iron and protein.

Avocado and Mango Salad—Makes 4–5 portions

2 Ripe avocados, lemon juice, 1 mango, 3 tbsp. Olive oil, 1 tsps. Wholegrain mustard, 2 tsps. Maple syrup, 2 tsps cider vinegar, shredded ice-berg Lettice, half a cucumber, 160 g of cooked chicken.

Mix the oil, mustard, vinegar and maple syrup together. Season with salt and pepper (optional). Shred the Lettice, mango and cucumber into small strips, place these into a large mixing bowl. Set aside. Cook the chicken in a little olive oil until cooked through (you can use chicken slices if preferred). Slice the avocado and drizzle with the lemon juice to prevent discolouration.

To Serve, place the mixed salad onto a plate, place avocado slices and cooked chicken slices—drizzle with the dressing before serving. This light lunch is high in protein, fibre, vitamin C, and beta-carotene. I would serve with a small bread roll and a small glass of juice.

Butternut Squash and Red Lentil Soup—Makes 4–6 portions

1 Butternut squash, 3 garlic cloves, 2 celery sticks, 1 large onion, 1 leek, sprig of thyme, a bay leaf, 20 g of red split lentils, 1 can of tomatoes, 2 litres of vegetable stock, 2 tbsp. Oil, crème fraiche to serve (optional).

Use a heavy-based pan, heat oil slightly and add chopped onions and celery, allow these to soften for about 5 min. Then add crushed garlic, chopped leak and cook further for 2 min. Add in chopped butternut squash, can of tomatoes, lentils, thyme and bay leaf. Mix well. Season with salt and pepper, then add the vegetable stock. Allow to cook on a low heat for about 10–15 min. Check the vegetables and lentils are cooked through, add additional water if necessary. Once the vegetables and lentils are cooked, blend the soup using a hand-held blender to a smooth consistency. Season to taste. Serve with a fresh roll of bread and a spoon of crème fraiche (optional). This soup is a source of protein, fibre, allicin, zinc, folic acid, fibre and potassium.

Slow Cooked Lamb with Steamed Spinach and Mash—Makes 4–6 portions

450 Lamb stewing lamb (you can an alternative cuts of lamb), 1 red onion, can of chickpeas, small piece of fresh ginger, 1 piece of garlic, 1 can chopped tomatoes, 1 tsps Mild Caribbean curry powder, pinch of salt, can of coconut milk.

Gently brown the meat in a pan, add a little oil if necessary, then place in a slow cooker or casserole dish. Dice the onion, ginger and garlic and lightly fry off in the pan, using up juices from the meat—transfer to the slow cooker. Add the tomatoes, curry powder, seasoning and mix well to combine the flavours. Add a little water if necessary. Cook in the slow cooker for about 4 h—check the meat is tender, then add the chickpeas and coconut milk. Stir well and cook for a further hour on a high setting. You can place in the oven if you prefer to cook through. Ensure the lamb is soft and tender.

For the Mash:

Peel and dice three large potatoes, boil until cooked through. Mash adding a little butter and milk. Ensure the texture is soft and creamy.

For the Spinach:

Place the spinach leaves in a steamer and steam for about 5 min, check the spinach is cooked and soft through, then rinse in cold water to retain the colour.

Serve the lamb with spinach and mash. Add a sauce over the lamb and mash. This dish is high in protein, iron, and vitamins K and C.

Warm Spicy Eggs and Wholemeal Pitta Bread

Ingredients: 2 medium sized eggs, half red onion (optional), 1 tsp of coconut fat, pinch of garam masala, pinch of Himalayan salt and ready-made pitta bread.

1. Whisk the eggs in a bowl then set aside. Heat the oil in a frying pan and add chopped red onion.
2. Allow the onion to cook for a couple of minutes until soft; then add the garam masala and eggs. Cook through on a gentle heat and continue to stir until the eggs are ready.
3. Serve the eggs with a warm pitta bread.

Eggs are a great source of protein, vitamin D, vitamin B-12, iron and selenium. The pitta bread is a good source of complex carbohydrates and fibre.

5.13   Reflection Points

- Reflect on your personal food beliefs and consider:
  - Think about how you could make changes to.
  - Whether there are any changes you could make to your nutrition and exercise to improve your health.
  - How easy or difficult do you think it would be to make changes? How to continually make changes to either maintain or improve nutritional status and physical activity?

References

Andro M, Squere P, Estivin S, Gentric A (2013) Anaemia and cognitive performances in the elderly: a systematic review. Eur J Neurol 20(9):1234–1240

Artaza-Artabe I, Sáez-López P, Sánchez-Hernández N, Fernández-Gutierrez N, Malafarina V (2016) The relationship between nutrition and frailty: effects of protein intake, nutritional supplementation, vitamin D and exercise on muscle metabolism in the elderly. A systematic review. Maturitas 93:89–99

Bauer J, Biolo G, Cederholm T, Cesari M, Cruz-Jentoft AJ, Morley JE, Phillips S, Sieber C, Stehle P, Teta D, Visvanathan R (2013) Evidence-based recommendations for optimal dietary protein intake in older people: a position paper from the PROT-AGE Study Group. J Am Med Dir Assoc 14(8):542–559

Beaudart C, Buckinx F, Rabenda V, Gillain S, Cavalier E, Slomian J, Petermans J, Reginster JY, Bruyère O (2014) The effects of vitamin D on skeletal muscle strength, muscle mass, and muscle power: a systematic review and meta-analysis of randomized controlled trials. J Clin Endocrinol Metabol 99(11):4336–4345

Beverly EA, Fitzgerald S, Sitnikov L, Ganda OP, Caballero AE, Weinger K (2013) Do older adults aged 60–75 years benefit from diabetes behavioral interventions? Diabetes Care 36(6):1501–1506

Bianchi L, Zuliani G, Volpato S (2013) Physical disability in the elderly with diabetes: epidemiology and mechanisms. Curr Diab Rep 13(6):824–830

Bollwein J, Volkert D, Diekmann R, Kaiser MJ, Uter W, Vidal K, Sieber CC, Bauer JM (2013) Nutritional status according to the mini nutritional assessment (MNA®) and frailty in community dwelling older persons: a close relationship. J Nutr Health Aging 17(4):351–356

Burd NA, Yang Y, Moore DR, Tang JE, Tarnopolsky MA, Phillips SM (2012) Greater stimulation of myofibrillar protein synthesis with ingestion of whey protein isolate v. micellar casein at rest and after resistance exercise in elderly men. Br J Nutr 108(6):958–962

Campbell N (2016) Innovations to support hydration care across health and social care. Br J Community Nurs 21:S24

Castro-Rodríguez M, Carnicero JA, Garcia-Garcia FJ, Walter S, Morley JE, Rodríguez-Artalejo F, Sinclair AJ, Rodríguez-Mañas L (2016) Frailty as a major factor in the increased risk of death and disability in older people with diabetes. J Am Med Dir Assoc 17(10):949–955

Cintra G, De Rezende NA, De Moraes EN, Cunha M, Torres HDG (2014) A comparison of survival, pneumonia, and hospitalization in patients with advanced dementia and dysphagia receiving either oral or enteral nutrition. J Nutr Health Aging 18(10):894

Corriere M, Rooparinesingh N, Kalyani RR (2013) Epidemiology of diabetes and diabetes complications in the elderly: an emerging public health burden. Curr Diab Rep 13(6):805–813

Deutz NE, Bauer JM, Barazzoni R, Biolo G, Boirie Y, Bosy-Westphal A, Cederholm T, Cruz-Jentoft A, Krznariç Z, Nair KS, Singer P (2014) Protein intake and exercise for optimal muscle function with aging: recommendations from the ESPEN Expert Group. Clin Nutr 33(6):929–936

Dominguez LJ, Barbagallo M (2017) The relevance of nutrition for the concept of cognitive frailty. Curr Opin Clin Nutr Metab Care 20(1):61–68

El-Sharkawy AM, Watson P, Neal KR, Ljungqvist O, Maughan RJ, Sahota O, Lobo DN (2015) Hydration and outcome in older patients admitted to hospital (The HOOP prospective cohort study). Age Ageing 44(6):943–947

García-Esquinas E, Graciani A, Guallar-Castillón P, López-García E, Rodríguez-Mañas L, Rodríguez-Artalejo F (2015) Diabetes and risk of frailty and its potential mechanisms: a prospective cohort study of older adults. J Am Med Dir Assoc 16(9):748–754

Goldberg LS, Altman KW (2014) The role of gastrostomy tube placement in advanced dementia with dysphagia: a critical review. Clin Interv Aging 9:1733

Greenberger C (2015 Jun) Enteral nutrition in end of life care: The Jewish Halachic ethics. Nurs Ethics 22(4):440–451

Heiland EG, Welmer AK, Wang R, Santoni G, Angleman S, Fratiglioni L, Qiu C (2016) Association of mobility limitations with incident disability among older adults: a population-based study. Age Ageing 45(6):812–819

Heisler M, Cole I, Weir D, Kerr EA, Hayward RA (2007) Does physician communication influence older patients' diabetes self-management and glycemic control? Results from the Health and Retirement Study (HRS). J Gerontol Ser A Biol Med Sci 62(12):1435–1442

Hong J, Kim J, Kim SW, Kong HJ (2017) Effects of home-based tele-exercise on sarcopenia among community-dwelling elderly adults: body composition and functional fitness. Exp Gerontol 87:33–39

Iwasa H, Masui Y, Gondo Y, Inagaki H, Kawaai C, Suzuki T (2008) Personality and all-cause mortality among older adults dwelling in a Japanese community: a five-year population-based prospective cohort study. Am J Geriatr Psychiatry 16(5):399–405

Kalyani RR, Metter EJ, Egan J, Golden SH, Ferrucci L (2015) Hyperglycemia predicts persistently lower muscle strength with aging. Diabetes Care 38(1):82–90

Van Kan GA, Vellas B (2011) Is the mini nutritional assessment an appropriate tool to assess frailty in older adults? J Nutr Health Aging 15(3):159–161

Kojima G, Taniguchi Y, Iliffe S, Walters K (2016) Frailty as a predictor of Alzheimer disease, vascular dementia, and all dementia among community-dwelling older people: a systematic review and meta-analysis. J Am Med Dir Assoc 17(10):881–888

Kumar V, Atherton P, Smith K, Rennie MJ (2009) Human muscle protein synthesis and breakdown during and after exercise. J Appl Physiol 106(6):2026–2039

Ley SH, Hamdy O, Mohan V, Hu FB (2014) Prevention and management of type 2 diabetes: dietary components and nutritional strategies. Lancet 383(9933):1999–2007

Lopez A, Cacoub P, Macdougall IC, Peyrin-Biroulet L (2016) Iron deficiency anaemia. Lancet 387(10021):907–916

Lu FP, Lin KP, Kuo HK (2009) Diabetes and the risk of multi-system aging phenotypes: a systematic review and meta-analysis. PLoS One 4(1):e4144

McCrow J, Morton M, Travers C, Harvey K, Eeles E (2016) Associations between dehydration, cognitive impairment, and frailty in older hospitalized patients: an exploratory study. J Gerontol Nurs 42(5):19–27

McClure R, Villani A (2017) Mediterranean diet attenuates risk of frailty and sarcopenia: new insights and future directions. JCSM Clin Rep 2(2):e00045

Moore EM, Ames D, Mander AG, Carne RP, Brodaty H, Woodward MC, Boundy K, Ellis KA, Bush AI, Faux NG, Martins RN (2014) Among vitamin B12 deficient older people, high folate levels are associated with worse cognitive function: combined data from three cohorts. J Alzheimers Dis 39(3):661–668

Morley JE (2012) Anorexia of aging: a true geriatric syndrome. J Nutr Health Aging 16(5):422–425

Ngandu T, Lehtisalo J, Solomon A, Levälahti E, Ahtiluoto S, Antikainen R, Bäckman L, Hänninen T, Jula A, Laatikainen T, Lindström J (2015) A 2 year multidomain intervention of diet, exercise, cognitive training, and vascular risk monitoring versus control to prevent cognitive decline in at-risk elderly people (FINGER): a randomised controlled trial. Lancet 385(9984):2255–2263

Park SW, Goodpaster BH, Strotmeyer ES, Kuller LH, Broudeau R, Kammerer C, De Rekeneire N, Harris TB, Schwartz AV, Tylavsky FA, Cho YW (2007) Accelerated loss of skeletal muscle strength in older adults with type 2 diabetes. Diabetes Care 30(6):1507–1512

Paul L, Selhub J (2017) Interaction between excess folate and low vitamin B12 status. Mol Aspects Med 53:43–47

Robinson S, Cooper C, Sayer AA (2012) Nutrition and sarcopenia: a review of the evidence and implications for preventive strategies. J Aging Res 2012, Article ID 510801, 6 p

Sala-Vila A, Díaz-López A, Valls-Pedret C, Cofán M, García-Layana A, Lamuela-Raventós RM, Castañer O, Zanon-Moreno V, Martinez-Gonzalez MA, Toledo E, Basora J (2016) Dietary marine ω-3 fatty acids and incident sight-threatening retinopathy in middle-aged and older individuals with type 2 diabetes: prospective investigation from the PREDIMED trial. JAMA Ophthalmol 134(10):1142–1149

Schrader E, Baumgartel C, Gueldenzoph H, Stehle P, Uter W, Sieber CC, Volkerf D (2014) Nutritional status according to Mini Nutritional Assessment is related to functional status in geriatric patients—independent of health status. J Nutr Health Aging 18(3):257

Serra-Prat M, Sist X, Domenich R, Jurado L, Saiz A, Roces A, Palomera E, Tarradelles M, Papiol M (2017) Effectiveness of an intervention to prevent frailty in pre-frail community-dwelling older people consulting in primary care: a randomised controlled trial. Age Ageing 46(3):401–407

de Souto Barreto P, Morley JE, Chodzko-Zajko W, Pitkala KH, Weening-Djiksterhuis E, Rodriguez-Mañas L, Barbagallo M, Rosendahl E, Sinclair A, Landi F, Izquierdo M (2016) Recommendations on physical activity and exercise for older adults living in long-term care facilities: a taskforce report. J Am Med Dir Assoc 17(5):381–392

Telenius EW, Engedal K, Bergland A (2015) Effect of a high-intensity exercise program on physical function and mental health in nursing home residents with dementia: an assessor blinded randomized controlled trial. PLoS One 10(5):e0126102

Volpato S, Bianchi L, Lauretani F, Lauretani F, Bandinelli S, Guralnik JM, Zuliani G, Ferrucci L (2012) Role of muscle mass and muscle quality in the association between diabetes and gait speed. Diabetes Care 35(8):1672–1679

Medicines and Older People with Diabetes: Beliefs, Benefits and Risks

Trisha Dunning

> *Poisons and medicine are often the same substance given with different intents*
>
> *(Peter Mere Latham, 19th-century English physician and educator).*

Key Points

- Most older people with diabetes use multiple medicines (polypharmacy).
- Polypharmacy can be thoughtful and appropriate or ad hoc and inappropriate.
- Medicine-related errors and adverse events are common causes of preventable hospital admissions for older people. Medicine-related adverse events also occur in hospital.
- Hypoglycaemia is the most significant adverse event associated with glucose lowering medicines and can occur at *any* blood glucose level.
- Medicine self-management becomes challenging with increasing age, functional, sensory and cognitive changes, access to health services and costs.
- Blood glucose monitoring can be a useful management guide if it reflects the action profile of the prescribed glucose lowering medicines.

6.1 Introduction

The purpose of this chapter is to discuss medicine management, especially the art of selecting and prescribing (personalising) medicines with older people with diabetes and sometimes with families. The chapter does not focus on prescribing information that is readily available in various medicine formularies, guidelines and algorithms. Table 6.1 outlines the classes of glucose lowering (GLM) medicines, their main actions and side effects and important issues to consider when deciding the GLM requirements with older people.

T. Dunning, A.M., M.Ed., Ph.D., R.N., C.D.E.
Centre for Quality and Patient Safety Research, Barwon Health Partnership,
Deakin University, Geelong, VIC, Australia
e-mail: trisha.dunning@barwonhealth.org.au;
trisha.dunning@deakin.edu.au

© Springer International Publishing AG, part of Springer Nature 2018
T. Dunning (ed.), *The Art and Science of Personalising Care with Older People with Diabetes*, https://doi.org/10.1007/978-3-319-74360-8_6

Table 6.1 Commonly used glucose lowering medicines and issues to consider when managing medicines with older people with diabetes

Medicine class	Main actions	Issues to consider
Metformin	Reduces hepatic glucose output. Alters the gut microbiome and contributes to blood glucose lowering effect.	Metformin is the most commonly used oral GLM especially in overweight people. Monitor renal function and adjust or cease medicines such as metformin if renal function declines, e.g. creatinine >150 mmol/L or eGFR < 30 mL/min/1.73 m squared. Metformin is associated with impaired absorption of vitamin B_{12} with long-term use and people with anaemia or peripheral neuropathy. hbA1c can be lower than actual levels in people with anaemia and is not a good indicator of metabolic control Supplements may be required. Metformin may also be contraindicated it the person is at risk of lactic acidosis, experiences gastrointestinal symptoms such as nausea and flatulence and has significant weight loss.
Sulphonylureas	Binds to beta cell receptors and triggers insulin release independently of glucose. Glucose stimulates insulin release (Chap. 1)	All sulphonylureas cause hypoglycaemia. Hypoglycaemia is a significant risk in older people and is associated with falls and trauma, changes in the myocardium and death. Sulphonylureas may be contraindicated if the person eats erratically and/or has renal or liver disease or acute weight loss because of the increased hypoglycaemia risk. Long-acting sulphonylureas are contraindicated in older people.
Alpha-glucosidase inhibitors.	Slow carbohydrate digestion and absorption form the gut and reduce post prandial blood glucose.	Gastrointestinal problems such as bloating and flatulence. They may have cardiovascular benefits.
Thiazolididones (TZD)	Sensitises tissues to insulin which enhances glucose entry into cells.	TZDs can be useful if the person has significant insulin resistance. They should not be used if the individual has liver and/or congestive heart failure TZD can cause oedema, which can cause discomfort and uncomfortable symptoms and limit function. Pioglitazone is associated with risk of bladder cancer and should not be prescribed for people diagnosed with bladder cancer. Risk of fractures in extremities, especially in women.

Table 6.1 (continued)

Medicine class	Main actions	Issues to consider
Incretins GLP-1 agonists and DPP-4 inhibitors	DPP-4 enhance endogenous GLP-1, and suppress glucagon suppression and enhance insulin secretion. GLP-1 agonists promote the same effects as DPP4 inhibitors. They also slow gastric emptying and increase satiety.	Combining GLP-1 and sulphonylurea increases the risk of hypoglycaemia. GLP-1 can cause nausea and weight loss and may be contraindicated in people at risk of weight loss. It may contribute to loss of muscle mass and frailty through weight loss. Both GLP-1 and DPP-4 have been associated with pancreatitis and may not be indicated in people with pancreatic disease. Should be stopped if they cause abdominal pain. They also help control hypertension. DPP-4 might cause heart failure in people with or at risk of cardiovascular disease and those with renal impairment.
Sodium-glucose cotransporter-2 inhibitors (SGLT-2)	Inhibit the SGLT-2 transporter exchange of sodium and glucose in the kidney and glucose is excreted in the urine. Some reduce systolic blood pressure and cardiovascular risk	May contribute to dehydration, dizziness that can cause electrolyte changes and increase the risk of ketoacidosis and the need for hospitalisation. SGLT-2-indicated ketoacidosis can occur without significant hyperglycaemia (euglycaemic ketoacidosis). Symptoms include dyspnoea, nausea, vomiting and abdominal pain. The medicine should be stopped if these symptoms develop. They are associated with urinary tract and genital infections and polyuria.
Insulin There are several types: Rapid-acting Short-acting Premixed insulins with differing proportions of rapid and intermediate or long-acting insulin Intermediate-acting Long-acting, which are often insulin analogues and cannot be mixed with other insulins	Is used to replace deficient endogenous insulin to keep blood glucose in the target range. Various dose regimens are used	Most people with T2DM eventually require insulin. Insulin can be combined with some other GLMs but that can complicate medicine self-care and add to the medicine-burden for older people. Insulin doses are easier to adjust than oral GLMs. Initiating insulin can reduce the medicine burden and simplify the medicine regimen but increases the hypoglycaemia risk. Injecting rapid-acting insulin when people eat rather than at fixed times might be an appropriate hypoglycaemia risk reduction strategy in palliative situations and individuals with dementia. Most insulin is 'human' insulin but animal insulins are still available in some countries and may not be appropriate for some people for religious reasons. Concentrated or high dose insulin is also available in some countries and can be used for people with severe insulin resistance

Generally, medicines, including GLMs, have contributed to reducing disease burden and reduced health service utilisation and increased morbidity and mortality. However, they also have adverse consequences that contribute to hospital admissions: more hospitalisations are due to diabetes, asthma and heart failure medicines than any other medicines (Australian Council Safety Quality Healthcare Standards (Australian Commission on Safety and Quality in Healthcare (ACSQHC) 2011).

People older than 65 years are at risk of adverse effects from a variety of medicines due to physiologic changes, polypharmacy and diabetes complications and other comorbidities, which complicate medicine choices and medicine self-care (Lim et al. 2017). Lim et al. (2017) also found increasing age, Indian ethnicity, male and a high number of comorbidities and supplement use were associated with increasing medicine use. Potential inappropriate medicine use and potential drug interactions were associated with polypharmacy and increased utilisation of health care.

Often, diabetes care focuses on the single condition 'diabetes', so-called 'silo care'. Thus, older people with diabetes often consult other HP specialists and disciplines, who might also provide 'silo care', and set the scene for uncoordinated care and polypharmacy. Diabetes can be overlooked when another comorbidity emerges or leads to a hospital admission. Most people over age 75 have several coexisting conditions and want to be treated as an individual and receive personalised coordinated care, even when they are frail and require more care than those who are not frail:

> I am not a collection of diseases hobbling around on a walker frame, wearing a nappy, worrying about falling and taking medicines for 'everything.' I need help to take my medicines. Do you know how difficult it is to take medicines when you are old?

Do you?
Some of the steps involved in taking medicines are:

- Having the medicines to take.
- Knowing, when, why and how to take them.
- Having sufficient vision to be able to read the package labels and any other medicines information.
- Opening the container, which requires on manual dexterity and eye-hand coordination.
- Removing medicines from the container.
- Being able to swallow oral medicines and/or inject insulin.
- Being able to check the accuracy of medicines prepacked in medicine dose aids.

These medicine tasks usually need to be repeated several times a day, which can disrupt life activities and be challenging to remember, especially when the individual has cognitive impairment or dementia. As indicated in Chap. 1, hypo- and hyperglycemia affect cognitive functions such as decision-making and problem-solving in the short term. These are key executive functions needed to manage medicines. Diet and physical activity remain important aspects of care, even when medicines are indicated, see Chap. 5, and dietary intake and timing of meals and food-medicine interactions need to be considered when planning care.

He who takes medicine and neglects diet wastes the skill of his doctors (Chinese proverb).

Almost all older people with diabetes require medicines to manage blood glucose and diabetes complications. Research suggests that 90% of people aged 65 years or older are prescribed at least one medicine and nearly 50% of older people are prescribed five or more medicines (Hilmer et al. 2013). These estimates do not include traditional and complementary medicines and therapies (T&CM) or self-prescribed over-the-counter medicines. People with type 2 diabetes (T2DM) often take an average of 7.4 medicines per day, range one to 25 in multiple doses at various times during the day (Dunning and Manias 2005). They also often take one or more antihypertensive agents, more than one GLM and/or insulin, and lipid lowering agents as well as other medicines.

Medicine choices and medicine self-management become more complex for older people because of functional, sensory and cognitive changes and social factors such as access to services and costs. Family members often assume some of the burden and help older people manage their medicines when they can no longer manage alone. However, family often do not always receive relevant medicine education and other information (Savage et al. 2012).

Medicine-self management requires people to understand their medicines and make important medicine-related decisions, in addition to the list of tasks described previously, often several times a day. Medicines self-management becomes increasingly burdensome with age and adds to the disease and treatment burdens (Rogers et al. 2017).

Medicine self-management involves:

- Consulting relevant prescribers to obtain prescriptions and having them filled.
- Informing health professionals about all the medicines they are taking, including T&CM.
- Having prescriptions filled.
- Taking the medicines 'as prescribed', see previous list.
- Monitoring their response to the medicine, e.g. monitoring blood glucose and ketones.
- Being able to recognise and manage medicine-related adverse events such as hypoglycaemia and hyperglycaemia, which is not as simple as it sounds because the 'text book' symptoms of these conditions change with duration of diabetes and diabetes complications such as neuropathy (Cryer et al. 2003).
- Consuming a healthy diet and having regular activity at times relevant to the action profile of their medicines.
- Being able to read, understand and apply medicines information.
- Actively seeking or clarifying information when needed.
- Attending regular health reviews and medicine reviews to assess medicine-related parameters such as HbA1c, lipids, and blood pressure.
- Navigating health services.

- Remembering to take the medicines, which is a common issue for many people, not only older people. Therefore, personalized medicine education for older people should include deciding cues with the individual to help them remember to take their medicines and information about what to do it they miss a dose or doses.

6.2   Cognitive Capacity to Self-Manage Medicines

Cognitive capacity refers to an individual's general learning ability, concentration, attention, visual perception, information processing, multi-tasking, executive functioning, reasoning, communication, planning, organising and emotional status (Glisky et al. 2001). Increasing age is not necessarily associated with cognitive decline. However, the cognitive functions most affected by age are attention and memory (Glisky et al. 2001), which are essential to diabetes self-care and medicine management. Family carers and other carers play a significant role assisting older people to manage their medicines at home.

Many carers have poor health. Stress, depression and cardiovascular disease are common; they often neglect their own self-care, and are at increased risk of dying (Family Caregiver Alliance 2010) and are often non-adherent to their own medicines (Shrank et al. 2011). Managing GLMs represents a significant burden. Family carers spend an average of 10.1 h per week managing oral GLMs and 14.1 h per week managing insulin compared to 6 h per week caring for people without diabetes. This significant burden of care is one reason families place older relatives in age care homes (Family Caregiver Alliance 2010).

Medicine management represents significant work and cognitive load and affects the individual's functioning and well-being. Diabetes and other endocrine disorders are independently associated with a higher likelihood of experiencing treatment burden (Sav et al. 2016). Significantly, high treatment burden is associated with higher HbA1c and inadequate self-care (Sav et al. 2016). Stopping unnecessary medicines, using non-medicine options and using combination medicines when possible are some ways to reduce the medicine burden (Dunning and Sinclair 2014).

However, HPs are taught to focus on achieving near normal blood glucose to meet guideline standards ('good control or tight control'), consequently, they often 'intensify treatment. Intensifying treatment includes using larger doses, more frequent doses and/or additional medicines; that is, add another GLM to the medicine regimen or initiate insulin in people with type 2 diabetes (T2DM), which further increases the medicine burden and associated workload for the individual as well as the risk of adverse events. It compromises adherence to the management plan and reduces the individual's physical and mental health and quality of life.

The American Diabetes Association recommended undertaking psychosocial assessments as part of personalising care, especially understanding the individual's care goals, preferences and priorities (Young-Hyman et al. 2016). Personalised care is described in Chaps. 2 and 3. Personalising care should involve assessing treatment burden as part of a comprehensive assessment, for example, using tools such the Patient Experience with Treatment and Self-Management (PETS) (Rogers et al. 2017). Alternatively, or in addition, HPs can ask the individual and/or family whether they are having any problems managing their medicines using non-judgmental language.

HPs need to understand the factors that affect medicine pharmacokinetics and pharmacodynamics, medicine adverse event profiles, beliefs about medicines, which can be influenced by culture, and be able to convey information in a manner suitable for older people/families using appropriate teaching methods and language to support older people's medicine self-management practices in a positive and affirming way. Negative, judgmental language is disempowering and leads to medicine non-adherence and suboptimal outcomes and was discussed in Chap. 1. Table 6.2 outlines some medicine-related information HPs can use to help older people and families manage their medicines safely.

In fact, people with diabetes Managing medicines is only one self-care task people with diabetes are expected to undertake and does not always take priority in people's lives. Older people have many unique ways of solving their medicine and other problems. For example:

I've run out of my insulin.

I'm sorry to hear that. I am happy to help you, but I cannot write a prescription. Can you see your GP?

I don't really want to do that. He was angry with me last time I ran out.

Do you run out of insulin very often?

Sometimes. Me and my dog are feeling pretty miserable this time though—thirst, weeing all over the place and we are so tired.

Can I check—you and your dog are both on insulin, but neither of you have had insulin for a while and now you are both feeling tired and weeing a lot.

Yes. We used up all my insulin then we used his insulin now we have no insulin left. I am really worried about Blackie, he is feeling awful. We always share everything, share our insulin.

The HP suggested the lady go to her vet on the way home to get some insulin for her dog and then to her GP to get herself some insulin. The lady's first concern was her dog's health. By putting the dogs' welfare first and accepting the lady's priorities and not lecturing her about her 'non-adherence' the HP was able to help the lady find a solution to her problem. She did visit the vet, then her GP and replaced her own and her dog's insulin. They both felt better after having insulin. Later the vet informed the HP '*she is my most non-compliant mother, she does this all the time!!*'

Table 6.2 outline of some of the factors associated with medicine-related adverse events derived from: The Australian Institute of Health and Welfare (2009), Stowasser et al. (2004); The Australian Commission on Safety and Quality in Health Care (Australian Commission on Safety and Quality in Healthcare (ACSQHC) 2011), Newman (2010)

• Older age: 30% of unplanned hospital admissions of older people involve medicine adverse events.
• People with serious health condition using five or more medicines regularly each day and more than 12 doses per day.
• Medicines with a narrow therapeutic index such as insulin.
• Recent transitions between care services.
• Discharge form hospital in the previous 4 weeks.
• Medicine regimen changes in the previous 3 months, especially when they are not documented on discharge summaries or communicated to other relevant HPs, the individual or family carers.
• Consulting several HPs.
• Traditional and complementary medicines (T&CM) use, especially when they do not disclose their T&CM use and when it is not documented on the medicine regimen.
• People with literacy and numeracy deficits.
• Administering medicines via the wrong route, which can be a HP, a person with diabetes or a family carer administration error.
• HP transcribing telephone medicine orders.
• HP distractions during medicine administration rounds.

6.3 Quality Use of Medicines

Quality Use of Medicines (QUM) (Commonwealth Department of Health and Aging 2002) encompasses all stages of the medicine process. QUM was initiated in Australia and is now used in several countries. QUM encompasses:

- Medicine regulation that includes assessing research evidence to determine the safety and benefit of medicines.
- Approving them for use.
- Manufacturing processes.
- Labelling.
- Marketing
- Storing and disposing of unused and out-of-date medicines.

HPs can use QUM to help older people with diabetes and families manage medicines; that is the clinical application of QUM is an important aspect of personalised care where it encompasses undertaking appropriate comprehensive assessments to decide whether medicines are actually indicated, which medicines would suit the individual, and any risks and benefits from individual medicines and medicines used in combination with other medicines.

A comprehensive assessment should include:

- Reviewing the medicine regimen and identifying medicines that are contra-indicated/should be used cautiously in older people, e.g. medicines on the

Beers Criteria, decide whether any medicine/s can be stopped before commencing another medicine using STOPP/START criteria (O'Mahony et al. 2015).

- Determining whether the person's health history includes any medicine alerts and/or red flags such as a medicine-related adverse event such as hypoglycaemia or allergies and cultural and religious concerns about medicines that contain animal products. A number of medicines contain products derived from animals, most commonly pork and beef (UK National Prescribing Centre 2004; Eldred et al. 2006)
- Undertaking relevant risk assessment such as hypoglycaemia risk and medicine-related adverse event risk (Dunning et al. 2013).
- Asking about complementary medicines use.
- Considering the hyperglycaemic effects of corticosteroids, antipsychotics and thiazide diuretics (diabetogenic medicines) in people with diabetes and older people with diabetes risk factors such as obesity, cardiovascular disease.
- Reviewing gastrointestinal, cardiovascular, liver and renal function, which are involved in medicine absorption, transport, metabolism and excretion, respectively.
- Assessing cognition and whether any cognitive deficits are temporary due to illness or likely to be permanent.
- Assessing risks related to specific medicines such as insulin and sulphonylureas, which cause hypoglycaemia. Hypoglycaemia is the most common insulin- and sulphonylurea-related adverse event in older people.
- Determining the individual's medicine self-management capacity and whether they need help to manage their medicines.
- Being aware that the individual's usual medicines can cause adverse events during intercurrent illnesses.

Then acting on the information derived from the assessment by:

- Stopping medicines where possible.
- Selecting and prescribing appropriate medicines, medicine doses in a dose form that suits the individual, e.g. liquids or patches if the individual has swallowing difficulties.
- Deciding how long the person needs to continue taking the medicine, which is usually ongoing for GLMs but might be a short course of an antibiotic for a urinary tract infection.
- Deciding how to monitor the effects of the medicine outcomes with the individual older person, e.g. blood glucose monitoring and pain relief.
- Documenting any errors and adverse events.
- Educating the older person and their family and other carers about how to take the medicines, how to store them and how to dispose of unused medicines, empty medicine container and medicine equipment such as syringes, needles and blood glucose test strips and finger prick lancets.
- How to recognise adverse events such as hypoglycaemia.

- Documenting and communicating relevant information such as management goals, triggers for medication review, when to stop medicines to other HPs, particularly when the individual consults several HPs and is transitioning among health services (Commonwealth Department of Health and Aging 2002). Care transitions are key adverse event points.

This list suggests managing medicines is a big responsibility for HPs and might also be burdensome for them as well as older people with diabetes and families.

6.4   Broad Medicine Care Aims and Strategies

Older people with diabetes should be involved in deciding medicine choices, care goals and care plans. Generally, the aim of prescribing medicines for older people with diabetes is to minimise the effects of hyperglycaemia, reduce glucose variability, and manage/prevent diabetes-related complications to ensure the individual is safe and has an acceptable quality of life.

Decisions need to be made about what constitutes a safe blood glucose and HbA1c range for the individual. The 'safe range' depends on the individual's functional category, disease trajectory and life expectancy (Dunning et al. 2013; IDF 2013). For example:

- Generally, a safe blood glucose range for older people on GLMs is between 6 and 11 mmol/L to reduce the risk of hypoglycaemia and its consequences such as falls and trauma.
- Healthy older people might be safe at HbA1c range 7–7.5%.
- Frail older people, people with dementia and those at the end of life might be safer at HbA1c range 8–8.5%.

6.5   Polypharmacy: The Good and the Not So Good

Polypharmacy refers to:

The use of a number of different medicines *possibly prescribed by different doctors and often filled in different pharmacies, by a patient who may have one or several health problems* Mosby's Medical Dictionary (2009).

Polypharmacy is not necessarily 'bad' if medicines are prescribed for a specific purpose with thought that results in appropriate medicine choices. However, polypharmacy is often 'unthoughtful' when new medicines are added to the existing medicine regimen without careful thought about the implications.

Polypharmacy could be classified thoughtful when HPs carefully consider recommendations in medicine titration algorithms and guidelines, because these decision aids were developed considering the several coexisting metabolic and other diabetes-related complications and comorbidities. However, algorithm-based decisions are only thoughtful, if they also include the effects on the individual and medicine burden and the person with diabetes is actively involved in making medicine-related decisions.

Some medicines cause serious adverse events that can lead to hospital admissions and are associated with significant morbidity and mortality (Green et al. 2007; Jenkins and Vaida 2007). Medicine-related adverse events occur *in* hospitals and aged care facilities and many are preventable (Roughead and Lexchin 2006; Jenkins and Vaida 2007). Insulin is commonly used to manage type 1 and type 2 diabetes. Insulin is classified as a high risk medicine because it carries a high risk of causing harm, even when it is used according to directions (Institute of Safe Medicine Practice (ISMP) 2008). Table 6.2 outlines some of the factors that lead to medicine-related adverse events.

As Paracelsus said, it is important to understand in order to use art and science well.

Medicine is not only a science; it is also an art. It does not consist of compounding pills and plasters; it deals with the very processes of life, which must be understood before they may be guided (Paracelsus 1493–1541).

6.6   Medicine-Self Management

Inappropriate medicine self-management affects outcomes such as blood glucose, lipid and blood pressure, which in turn affect function and quality of life. Medicine self-management is complex: the individual needs to learn and undertake complex medicine-specific self-care behaviours. Managing medicines can be particularly challenging for older people and they often need very simple direct messages, as the following anecdote shows.

Please help the doctor told me to take one of these tablets three times daily. I do not know what that means.

What three times?

Daily means once every day to me. If I was supposed to take them three time a day I should have been told that and told times to take them.

For a HP perspective the directions are clear—the man was told to take the medicine three times daily. The word 'daily' confused him.

I worried that I might take them too close together and kill myself too far apart and not they would wear off, so I played it safe and did not take them.

Various factors affect people with diabetes' ability to understand information: these include low health literacy and numeracy and lower socioeconomic status. However, often the reason they do not understand is because the information is ambivalent and unclear (Davis et al. 2009) as the man's story shows. The man's story is not an isolated event; people do not receive the medicine information they need to manage medicines safely from HPs (Dunning and Manias 2005).

The man was labelled non-compliant by another HP and sent for 'to be sorted out and some diabetes education'. Was he non-compliant or non-adherent OR did he make the best decision with the information he had at the time and then try to clarify the directions? Will the label be noted in his medical record and affect HP's perceptions of him in the future?

6.7   Compliance: A Modern 'no-no Label'—Or Is It?

Several diabetes position statement on language advocate avoiding the label 'compliant' and 'non-compliant' (Diabetes Australia 2011; IDF 2013; Dunning et al. 2017; Dickinson et al. 2017) because these words have evolved from their original meaning over time and now represent wayward, even bad behaviour (bad people). However, the word compliance consists of three inter-related concepts: acceptance, adherence and persistence.

Acceptance concerns an individual making an informed choice to take a medicines to improve or maintain their health (World Health Organisation (WHO) 2003). The man in the anecdote accepted he needed the medicine and had his prescription filled but he made an informed choice not take the medicine because the medicine self-management directions he received were not clear.

Adherence refers to whether the individual follows their medicine regimen (Cramer et al. 2007); the man did not follow the 'directions', but he had a logical reason for not taking the medicine that he based on his assessment of his personal risk. He sought advice to clarify the 'directions'. The HP should have checked to make sure the man understood his or her directions. One method of checking for understanding is to ask the individual to repeat the information back to the HP. That strategy might *not* have resulted in a different outcome if the man repeated *I am to take the medicine three times daily.* The direction would still be confusing for the man, but his response would have satisfied the HP.

Persistence refers to continuing to take the course of medicine from the time it is commenced to the time it is to be discontinued (Cramer et al. 2007). Some medicines such as insulin in type 1 diabetes are required for life; thus, we do not expect the person with type 1 to stop taking insulin, even temporarily. People with type 2 diabetes often require insulin for a short time, for example, during surgery and infections.

Optimal compliance is difficult to define. It probably includes one or all of acceptance, adherence and persistence that achieves relevant outcomes such as blood glucose in the individual's target range. The important issue is that the safe target range might vary among individuals, and the target ranges should be personalised.

In order to achieve understanding and make shared decisions, the individual, family and the HP need to be able to understand medicines and other relevant information and be informed about all the available options and their risks and benefits. HPs need to understand and accept that the individual's medicine beliefs and attitudes and behaviours may be different from their own. Shared decision-making is discussed in Chaps. 2 and 3. If a shared decision cannot be reached, the HP's preferred outcome might not to be achieved (Cramer et al. 2007)—the person with diabetes' might! Then again, it might not. It is important to understand factors from the various decision-makers' perspectives: the individual, families and HPs. The following information about various perspectives was compiled from the authors' various research and clinical experience over past 20 years.

6.8 People with Diabetes' Perspectives About Medicines

Understanding the person with diabetes' perspective is essential to enable the HP to help the person decide which medicine/s and medicine regimen is likely to suit their health needs without increasing the medicine self-management burden. People with diabetes consider many things when making decisions about medicines but they might not share them with HPs unless the HP asks. These include

- Cost.
- The side effects. Hypoglycaemia is a particular concern for many people who take insulin.
- Their capacity to remember to take the medicines and fit their medicine taking into their daily routines and to balance competing demands.
- Believing they are not sick—'only sick people take medicines'.
- The stigma associated with injecting insulin and monitoring blood glucose in public.
- How long they will need to keep taking the medicine.
- Medicine burden.
- Cultural customs and beliefs.

6.9 Health Professional's Perspectives

HPs generally base their decision to prescribe medicines and decide doses on different parameters from people with diabetes:

- A physical and mental assessment: but they do not always explore the individual's medicine-beliefs and attitudes in detail or their self-care capacity and often have time constraints during consultations.
- The information family carers and other HPs provide.
- Their preferences for specific medicines, which are influenced by a number of factors including pharmaceutical representatives providing prescribing information and lectures, reading and consulting other colleagues.
- Available decision-aids such as medicine formularies and diabetes guidelines.
- Their previous experience managing diabetes and its treatment.
- Concerns about multiple prescribers being involved and the risks associated with inadequate communication among prescribers and dispensers.

6.10 Family Care's Perspective of their Medicine-Management Role

Family often provide a significant amount of unpaid care and assume part or all of the care burden for older people with diabetes with physical and cognitive deficits. Carers can be adult children, grandchildren or are old and taking medicines themselves. Family carers are not always given education to help them in their carer role. For example, we found husbands and wives caring for their relatives with diabetes receiving palliative care were very distressed and unsure about their knowledge and ability to help their relative with diabetes perform self-care activities such as injecting insulin and blood glucose monitoring (Savage et al. 2012).

The stress of caring for an older relative may mean they neglect their own health. Thus, carers might need education about their own medicines and about how to fit medicine management into their other personal and care-giving responsibilities.

Caregiving activities include:

- Being prepared for anything.
- Being flexible and adaptable so they could manage 'if something happens'.
- Having regular contact with the individual to prevent problems or identify them early and seek help early.
- Helping the individual attend HP appointments, with activities of daily living and instrumental activities of daily living, which might include taking them to activities such as rehabilitation to help regain function.

Decisions become more complex in palliative and end of life situations when the individual cannot make decisions, especially when they are being cared for at home (Palliaged 2017). Concerns in this setting are:

- Having help to deliver care and to share the burden.
- Being anxious about the quality and usefulness of the care they provide.
- Having access to support for HPs and other family and carers.
- Being able to maintain relationships, especially where the care recipient is a spouse.
- Worry about supporting family when the individual dies.
- Worry about the responsibility for administering medicines and monitoring symptoms.

Family carers also report benefits such as finding meaning and personal growth in caring.

6.11 Medicine Adherence and Optimal Health Outcomes?

If people do not take their medicines, they will not 'work'. Adherence has a positive effect on outcomes (Di Matteo et al. 2002; Simpson et al. 2006). Di Matteo et al. (2002) analysed 63 studies and found adherence reduced the risk of no outcome or an inadequate outcome by 26% compared with non-adherence. The DCCT (1993) and UKPDS (1998) demonstrated lower in HbA_{1c}, which were partly due to medicines.

However, outcomes also depend on the pharmacodynamics of the individual's medicines, which in turn is affected by individual factors such as the person's age gender, physical and mental health and pharmacogenetics. In addition, changing

Table 6.3 Some factors that could alert HPs to individuals are at risk of medicine non-adherence

- Results of risk assessments for possible medicine non-adherence.
- Older age, cultural and other medicine beliefs, functional deficits.
- Cognitive changes especially to executive functions such as problem-solving, decision-making and remembering to take their medicines. These can be temporarily affected by hypo- and hyperglycaemia.
- Changes in HbA_{1c}, blood lipids and blood pressure.
- Prescriptions are not filled.
- The person misses scheduled appointments.
- Recent admission to hospital or ED.
- Depression.
- Lack of support and/or financial constraints.
- New problems emerge, e.g. pain, nausea, vomiting or hypoglycaemia
- Several coexisting comorbidities.
- Difficulty undertaking usual activities of daily living, e.g. opening medicine containers.
- Vision and/or hearing deficits, which can result in social isolation, not keeping HP appointment and miscommunication.
- Coping, problem-solving, self-esteem and interpersonal skill, deficits, which might indicate changes in cognition.
- Literacy and numeracy deficits.
- Specific medicine-related factors such as:
  - belief the medicine will not be beneficial
  - medicines that are not aligned with cultural or individual health beliefs.
  - unable or unwilling to answer questions about medicines self-care.
  - missing doses, inappropriately adjusting doses, stop medicines without advice, crush or later dose forms in appropriate ways.

medicine dose forms can affect duration of action and bioavailability. For example, crushing long-acting dose forms of metformin and inappropriately cutting medicines in half because of cost.

HP should ask about factors that could affect medicine management, some of which are outlined in Tables 6.2 and 6.3 some risk factors for medicine non-adherence.

Determining medicine adherence might be best achieved using a combination of methods, given it is a multifaceted concept. Some commonly used clinical monitoring methods include:

- Physiological measures as:
  - HbA_{1c}, blood glucose, blood lipids, blood pressure
  - blood and/or urine medicine levels
  - presence or absence of symptoms such as pain, thirst and polyuria, angina.
- Physical assessment and observation.
- Self-report from the individual and/or their carers monitoring records, which are often maintained on mobile phones but some people still use written diaries/record books, e.g. some people record their medicines use in their blood glucose diaries.

- Monitoring systems that compares actual and expected prescription refills according to the dose regimen (Pharmacy Guild of Australia 2010), which are more often used in medicines research than as clinical monitoring processes.
- Medicine tools, which have clinical and research applications, for example:
  - Brief Medicines questionnaire (BMQ)
  - Beliefs about Medicines Questionnaire (BaMQ)
  - Medicines Adherence Report Scale (MARS).

People with diabetes often use T&CM for various reasons and not necessarily to manage blood glucose.

6.12   Traditional and Complementary Medicines and Therapies

More than 50% of the populations of many countries use T&CM including people with diabetes (Egede et al. 2002; Dunning 2003; Manya et al. 2012). Most T&CM use is self-initiated but some people with diabetes consult T&CM practitioners. Some reasons people with diabetes use T&CM are to improve their general wellbeing and quality of life by managing pain, stress, and intercurrent illness and because 'they treat the whole person'.

Therefore, HPs need to ask about T&CM use, include T&CM medicines in the medicine regimen and understand that there is a growing evidence base for some T&CM. For example, Tai Chi is recommended to build muscle strength and flexibility and help reduce the risk of falls (Li et al. 2005).

6.13   Strategies HPs Can Use to Help Older People with People Take Their Medicines to Achieve Optimal Outcomes

Table 6.4 lists some strategies HPs can use to reduce medicine-related adverse events. However, The World health Organisation (WHO) (2003) indicated that fewer than 50% of strategies used to improve people's medicine adherence actually worked. HPs' relationship with and personalising medicine education with older people with diabetes and families can make a significant difference to the way individuals manage their medicines, and therefore, health outcomes. Personalising medicine education and management involves discussing the factors that make it difficult/easier for the individual to manage their medicines and providing relevant information in a format that suits the person's learning style (Williams et al. 2008).

HPs should also reflect on their medicine-related experiences beliefs and behaviours and ask themselves whether they adhere to their medicines regimen 100% of the time. They can also engage people with diabetes and family carers in discussions about medicines beliefs and self-management to help them develop medicine management plan that works for them providing appropriate medicine education.

Table 6.5 lists some important information that can help people with diabetes and families manage their medicines safely. Information is available in various mediums and HPs need to consider the individual's literacy and numeracy skills when

Table 6.4 Strategies and processes HPs can use to reduce medicine adverse events derived from Rommers et al. (2007); Wolfstadt et al. (2008); Dooley et al. (2011); Fowler and Rayman (2010) and the National Heart Foundation Australia (National Heart Foundation of Australia (NHFA) 2011)

- Asses the individual's risk of non-adherence: HP-related, individual factors, the situation and environment and family carer-related.
- Quality use of medicines and pharmacovigilance and regular medicine reviews to reduce polypharmacy. Medicine reviews might need to be undertaken frequently in older people, e.g. every hospital admission and change in health status.
- Follow quality and safety standards and guidelines.
- Use clinical decision support tools and systems to personalise care.
- Check any automated alert and red flag systems in use.
- Educate self, other HPs and people with diabetes and family carers.
- Consult pharmacists, medication safety committees and medicine review programmes for advice when needed.
- Effectively communicate with other HPs, people with diabetes and family carers when undertaking discharge planning from hospital.

Table 6.5 Information about medicines that can be included in medicine education to help older people with diabetes/families manage their medicines safely and effectively

- The name of the medicine including the name of the active ingredient in the medicine.
- Some people worry about taking generic medicines, explain what they are can help allay their concerns.
- What the medicine is for.
- How the medicine works.
- When to take the medicine.
- Any precautions with respect to food and exercise.
- How to take the medicine, e.g. insulin injection technique.
- How to store medicines including when travelling.
- The *individual's* likelihood of experiencing medicine-related side effects, how recognize a side effect and how to manage a side effect.
- Information about how to read the medicine label, not just when to take the medicine but information about the incipients, fillers, colourants and animal products in medicines because some people are allergic to or have cultural and religious reasons for not wanting to take medicines containing these additions.
- Use a system to highlight the differences between medicines that have similar names.
- How to dispose of unused medicines and related equipment.
- What cues or products could help the individual remember to take their medicines.
- What to do if they miss a dose/doses.
- When and how to stop taking such medicines prescribed for a specific time period (course).
- Who to contact for advice and how to contact them.
- How to find reliable information about medicines on the internet that meets standards in the 'Hon Code' (http://www.healthconnect.org/HONcode?conduct.html.

The information must be adapted to each individual older person's needs providing verbal and other information. Memory aids such as medicine dose aids, dose reminders, and mobile telephone alarms can be useful for older people who 'forget' to take their medicines n a regular basis.

Undertaking regular comprehensive medicine reviews is an essential aspect of care. Medicine reviews can be undertaken before prescribing a new medicine, any change in health or functional status and at key transitions such as admission to an aged care home. Undertaking medicine reviews in the individual's home can be very informative, provided it is done respectfully and sensitively.

6.14 Pharmacogenomics and Precision Medicine: The Way of the Future?

Genomics is beginning to change health care and the ability to influence health for the individual by understanding the nature of disease and the way medicines act at a molecular level (Cheek et al. 2015). The term precision medicine is used to refer to the ability to develop therapeutic interventions for specific individuals and the disease/s they have. The term pharmacogenomics encompasses the role of the whole genome in medicine responses. Pharmacogenetics generally refers to the role of single genes in medicine responses.

Three main classes of genes that influence how genes interact with a specific medicine are described:

1. Medicine metabolising pharmacogenetics—the role of variations in human genes that code for enzymes involved in metabolising the medicines that can activate or inactivate the medicine (Evrard and Mbatchi 2012)
2. Medicine-transporter pharmacogenetics—the role of variation in human genes that code for membrane transporters that transport medicines into or out of cells (Sissung et al. 2014)
3. Medicine-target pharmacogenetics—the role of variation in human genes that code for the medicine target or other proteins associated with the biochemical or regulatory medicine pathway (Johnson 2011).

Pharmacogenomics and pharmacogenetics are likely to influence diabetes medicine options in the future and is likely to reduce individual risks of adverse medicine and maximise their benefits. It will enable HPs to understand which medicines are affected by people of different ethnic groups (Yasuda 2016).

Diabetes-related pharmacogenetics shows sulphonylurea sensitivity in people with HNF1A Maturity Onset Diabetes in the Young (MODY) and in people with T2DM with reduced function at alleles at CY2CP. The latter leads to reduced sulphonylurea metabolism. Other MODY genetic variations lead to severe intolerance of Metformin (Pearson 2016). These genetic discoveries have enabled the various MODY genetic variants to be treated and improved outcomes for people with MODY.

The many genetic determinates of human ageing are also under study. Ageing is a major determinant of functional, independence and dignity. Genetic studies are underway to develop medicines that target ageing itself to reverse the pathogenesis of several diseases at the same time (Mallikarjun and Swift 2016).

These findings highlight the complex interacting associations between genes, disease processes and the individual's environment and personal factors such as beliefs and attitudes that will shape our understanding of personalised care in the future.

6.15 Chapter Summary

Medicine self-management is complex and challenging. HPs can play a key role helping older people with diabetes manage their medicines appropriately by engaging with the individual to determine and understand their beliefs about and experience of medicines, which will help put their medicine-related behaviours into perspective. The terms adherence and non-adherence are descriptors that mean many different things to HPs, people with diabetes and their carers. However, the terms should not be used as judgmental labels.

I thought carefully about using the terms 'take', 'use', and 'administer to refer to the act of 'taking a medicine'. I used 'take' in most places in the text but 'use' in some places to be consistent with the literature. To me, take refers to oral routes, 'use' can refer to any route as c administer, but the latter sound more like a HP word. One rarely hears a person with diabetes say 'I administered my insulin'.

6.16 Reflection Points

Think about your personal medicines beliefs and experiences and consider:

- How they affect the way you discuss medicines with older people with diabetes.
- Think about an event that shaped your medicine-related beliefs.
- Consider how you will engage and support family helping older people with diabetes manage their medicines.

References

Australian Commission on Safety and Quality in Healthcare (ACSQHC) (2011) National Safety and Quality Health Service Standards. ACSQHC, Canberra, pp 34–39

Australian Institute of Health and Welfare (AIHW) (2009) Australian hospital statistics 2007–8. AIHW, Canberra

Cheek D, Basshore L, Brazeau D (2015) Pharmacogenomic and implications for nursing practice. J Nurs Scholarsh 47(6):496–504

Commonwealth Department of Health and Aging (2002) The quality use of medicines. Commonwealth Department of Health and Aging, Canberra

Cramer J, Roy A, Burrell A, Fairchild C, Fuldeore M, Ollendorf D, Wong P, International Society for Pharmacoeconomics for Outcomes Research Working Group (2007) Medication compliance and persistence: terminology and definitions. Value Health 11(1):4447

Cryer P, Davis S, Shamoon H (2003) Hypoglycaemia in diabetes. Diabetes Care 26(6):1902–1912. www.health.gov.au/internet/main/publishing.nsf/content/nmp-**quality**.htm

Davis T, Federman A, Bass P, Jackson R et al (2009) Improving patient understanding of prescription drug label instructions. J Gen Intern Med 24:57–62

Di Matteo M, Giordani P, Lepper H, Croghan T (2002) Patient adherence and medical treatment outcomes: a meta-analysis. Med Care 40(9):794–811

Diabetes Australia. (DA) (2011) A new language for diabetes: improving communication with and about people with diabetes. DA, Canberra

Diabetes Control and Complications Trial Research Group (1993) The effect of intensive treatment of diabetes on the progression of long term complications of insulin dependent diabetes. N Engl J Med 329:977–986

Dickinson J, Guzman S, Melinda D et al (2017) The use of language in diabetes care and education. Diabetes Care. care.diabetesjournals.org/content/early/2017/09/26/dci17-0041

Dooley M, Wiseman M, McRae A et al (2011) Reducing potentially fatal errors associated with high doses of insulin: a successful multifaceted multidisciplinary prevention strategy. Br Med J. https://doi.org/10.1136/bmjqs.2010.049668

Dunning T (2003) Complementary therapies and diabetes. Complement Ther Nurs Midwifery 9:74–80

Dunning T, Manias E (2005) Medication knowledge and self-management by people with Type 2 diabetes. Aust J Adv Nurs 11:172–181

Dunning T, Sinclair S (2014) Glucose lowering medicines and older people with diabetes: the importance of comprehensive assessments and pharmacovigilance. J Nurs Care 3(3):1–9

Dunning T, Savage S, Duggan N. (2013) The McKellar guidelines for managing older people with diabetes.in residential and other care settings. http://www.adma.org.au/clearinghouse/doc_details/133-the-mckellar-guidelines-for-managing-older-people-with-diabetes-in-residential-and-other-care-settings_9dec2013.html

Dunning T, Speight J, Bennett C (2017) Language, the 'diabetes restricted code/dialect,' and what it means for people with diabetes and clinicians. Diabetes Educ 47(1):18–26

Egede L, Xiaobou Y, Zheng D, Silverstein M (2002) The prevalence and pattern of complementary and alternative medicine use in individuals with diabetes. Diabetes Care 25:324–329

Eldred B, Dean A, McGuire T, Nash A (2006) Vaccine components and constituents: responding to consumer concerns. Med J Aust 2184(4):170–175

Evrard A, Mbatchi L (2012) Genetic polymorphisms of drug metabolizing enzymes and transporters. The long way from bench to bedside. Curr Top Mol Chem 12(15):1720–1729

Family Caregiver Alliance (2010) http://www.caregiver.org/caregiver/jsp/content_node.jspp?nodeid=1822

Fowler D. Rayman G. (2010) Safe and effective use of insulin in hospitalised patients. National Health Service London. http://www.diabetes.nhs.uk/document.php?o=1040. Accessed Jan 2011

Glisky E, Rubin S, Davidson S (2001) Source memory in older adults: an encoding or retrieving problem. J Exp Psychol 27(5):1131–1146

Green J, Hawley J, Rask K (2007) Is the number of prescribing physicians an independent risk factor for adverse drug events in an elderly outpatient population? Am J Geriatr Pharmacother 5(1):31–39

Hilmer S, Gnijidic D, Le Couteur D (2013) Thinking through the medication list. Aust Fam Physician 12:924–928

Institute of Safe Medicine Practice (ISMP) 2008. www.ismp.org. Accessed Jan 2011.

International Diabetes Federation (IDF) (2013) Language philosophy. www.idf.org

Jenkins R, Vaida A. (2007) Simple strategies to avoid medication errors. AAFP http://www.aafp.org/fpm/2007/0200p41.html. Accessed Dec 2009.

Johnson J (2011) Drug target pharmacogenetics. Am J Pharmacogenomics 4:315–322

Li F, Harmer P, Fisher J et al (2005) Tai chi and fall reduction in older adults: a randomized controlled trial. J Gerontol: Med Sci 60A(2):187–194

Lim L, McStea M, Chung W et al (2017) Prevalence, risk factors and health outcomes associated with polypharmacy among urban community-dwelling older adults in multi-ethnic Malaysia. PLoS One. https://doi.org/10.1371/journal.pone.0173466

Mallikarjun V, Swift J (2016) Therapeutic manipulation of ageing: repurposing old dogs and discovering new tricks. EBioMedicnine. https://doi.org/10.1016/j.ebiom.2016.11.o2o

Manya K, Champion B, Dunning T (2012) The use of complementary and alternative medicine among people living with diabetes in Sydney. BMC Complement Altern Med. https://doi.org/10.1166/1472-6882-12-2

Mosby's Medical Dictionary (2009) 8th ed. Elservier.

National Heart Foundation of Australia (NHFA) (2011) Improving Adherence in cardiovascular care. NHFA

Newman B. (2010) Safety first. Nursing Rev 26

O'Mahony D, O'Sullivan D, Byrne S et al (2015) STOPP/START criteria for potentially inappropriate prescribing in older people: version 2. Age Ageing 44(2):213–218. https://doi.org/10.1093/ageing/afu145

Palliative Care—palliAGED (2017). https://www.palliaged.com.au/tabid/4338/Default.aspx

Pearson E (2016) Personalized medicine in diabetes: the role of 'omics' and biomarkers. Diabet Med 13(6):712–717

Rogers E, Yost K, Rosedahl J et al (2017) Validating the patient experience with treatment self-management (PETS), a patient-reported measure of treatment burden, in people with diabetes. Patient Rel Outcome Meas 8:143–156

Rommers M, Teepe-Twiss I, Guchelaar H-J (2007) Preventing adverse drug events in hospital practice: an overview. Pharmacepidemiol Drug Saf 16:1129–1135

Roughead E, Lexchin J (2006) Adverse drug events: counting s not enough, action is needed. Med J Aust 184(7):315–316

Sav A, Whitty J, McMillan S et al (2016) Treatment burden and chronic illness: who is most at risk? Patient 9(6):559–569

Savage S, Dunning T, Duggan N, Martin P (2012) The experiences and care preferences of people with diabetes at the end of life. J Hospice Palliative Care Nurs. https://doi.org/10.1097/NJH.0601e3184bdb39

Shrank W, Libeman J, Fischer M, Kiabuk E, Girdish C, Curtrona S, Brennan T, Chudhry N (2011) Are caregivers adherent to their own medications? J Am Pharm Assoc 51(4):492–498

Simpson S, Eurich D, Sadjeedp S, Ross I, Varney J, Johnson J (2006) A meta-analysis of the association between adherence to drug therapy and mortality. Br Med J 333:15–18

Sissung T, Goey A, Ley A et al (2014) Pharmacogenetics of membrane transporters: a review of current approaches. Methods Mol Biol 1175:91–120

Stowasser D, Allison Y, O'Leary Karen M (2004) Understanding the medicine management pathway. J Pharmacol Pract Res 34:293–296

The Pharmacy Guild of Australia (2010) Medindex: a medicine compliance indicator. The Pharmacy Guild of Australia, Canberra. http://www.medsindex.com.au

United Kingdom National Prescribing Centre (2004) Task Force on Medicines Partnership. Drugs of porcine origin and their clinical alternatives. An introductory guide; March 2004. Available from: http://www.mcb.org.uk/uploads/PBEnglish.pdf

United Kingdom Prospective Study (UKPDS 33, 34) (1998) Intensive blood glucose control. Lancet 352(837–853):854–865

Williams A, Manias E, Walker R (2008) Interventions to improve medication adherence in people with multiple chronic conditions: a systematic review. J Adv Nurs 63(2):132–143

Wolfstadt J, Gurwitz J, Field T, Lee M, Kalkar S, Wu W, Rochon P (2008) The effect of computerized physician order entry and clinical decision support on the rates of adverse drug events: a systematic review. J Gen Intern Med 23(4):451–458

World health Organisation (WHO) (2003) Adherence to long-term therapies: evidence for action. WHO, Geneva

Yasuda S, Zhang L, Huang S-M (2016) The role of ethnicity in variability in response to drugs: focus on clinical pharmacology. Stud Nat Pharmacol. http://www.tda.gov.downlods/Drugs/ScienceResearch/.../UCM0865502.pdf

Young-Hyman D, de Groot M, Hill-Briggs E et al (2016) Psychosocial care for people with diabetes: a position statement of the American Diabetes Association. Diabetes Care 29(12):2126–2140

Older People with Diabetes and Life Transitions

Bodil Rasmussen

> *Hold still. stay there. tease back the layers. you are in the space between your comfort zone and infinity. you want to hide. not be seen. not be open. not be vulnerable. But you have to. there are two ways to do this—soft and gentle or fast and hard. both will get you to the other side, if you let them.*
>
> *(Jeanette LeBlanc).*

Key Points

- Transitions are an important part of life from infancy to older age.
- Not all transitions are negative, they can represent an opportunity to enhance the person's quality of life.
- Salutogenesis stresses the importance of starting by considering how health is created and maintained rather than focusing on the negative aspects of illness and disorder.
- Social and psychological support are vital to encourage older people to manage diabetes and it is meaningful to them.

7.1 Introduction

The purpose of chapter seven is to address the impact of diabetes on usual life transitions in older age. Healthy ageing is a lifelong process that evolves through the lifespan from pre-conception, infancy, adolescence, and young adulthood into old age. Lifespan is usually understood to be the duration of a person's life from conception to the end of life (Kail and Cavanaugh 2018).

From a life course perspective, old age, 65 and older can be considered as the 'last season', or the third age, but reaching the age of 65 is not the last transition. Increasingly, we also talk about 'the fourth age' or 'the oldest old' to refer to people aged 85 and older. Life course in this context means the social aspect of the lifespan

B. Rasmussen
Western Health Partnership, Deakin University, Burwood Campus, VIC, Australia
e-mail: bodilr@deakin.edu.au

© Springer International Publishing AG, part of Springer Nature 2018
T. Dunning (ed.), *The Art and Science of Personalising Care with Older People with Diabetes*, https://doi.org/10.1007/978-3-319-74360-8_7

involving biological, social, and psychological processes that lead to planned or unplanned life transitions and/or events Koelen et al. 2017).

Older people are often viewed as passive and frail, even though in reality a substantial number are quite resilient and actively manage the challenges they face as part of the ageing process (Koelen et al. 2017; Nilson et al. 2010; Tan et al. 2013). With increasing age, many changes occur in the social environment as a result of retirement and the loss of the usual role, death of a spouse, death of family members and friends, and the onset of age-related sensory loss and mobility problems. Other transitions in older age might be admission to an aged care facility, which might involve grief and distress, stopping driving triggering lack of independence and autonomy, or the need for palliative care or end-of-life care.

Psychosocial stress, the ability to adjust to change and coping ability influences a person's self-care potential and for people with diabetes metabolic control, and impacts on clinical outcomes and mental health (Polonsky et al. 2005). Transitions are a familiar concept in developmental, stress and adaptation theories (Schlossberg et al. 1995).

The theory of medical sociologist, Antonovsky (1979, 1987a, b), which emphasises health and illness transitions, encompasses life transitions. Transitions and change in health status can be difficult, but they can also represent an opportunity to enhance quality of life (Antonovsky 1987a, b; Bridges 2001, 2002; Kralik and van Loon 2007; Rasmussen et al. 2007). Healthy ageing comprises wellness and quality of life constructs. Antonovsky's theory (1979, 1987a, b) is, therefore, particularly relevant to transitions in older people because it emphasises the wellness and quality of life aspects for people going through transitions. It also fits in with the current focus on flourishing in older age and restorative care (healthy ageing) strategies being adopted in many countries (Chap. 1).

7.1.1 The Sense of Coherence Construct

Approaches to health can either focus on the origins of health (salutogenic) or origins of disease (pathogenic) according to Antonovsky (1987a, b, 1991, 1993). The word 'salutogenesis' comes from the Latin *salus* = health and the Greek *genesis* = origin. Antonovsky developed the term from his studies of 'how people manage stress and stay well' (Antonovsky 1987a, b). He observed that stress is ever-present, but not all individuals have negative health outcomes in response to stress. Some people achieve health despite their exposure to potentially disabling stress factors.

7.1.1.1 Sense of Coherence and Salutogenesis
The sense of coherence (SOC) theory refers to people's different abilities to deal with challenges. SOC is a theoretical construct to explain why some individuals fall ill after a stressful situation and others do not. It involves:

- A global orientation of the individual to communicate and endure dynamic feelings of confidence triggered by stimuli in their internal and external environments in the course of living.

- How predictable and explicable the changes are, as well as whether resources are available to individuals to meet the demands posed by these stimuli.
- How these demands are perceived, for example, being challenged, being worthy of investment and engagement. (Antonovsky 1979, 1987a, b)

Salutogenesis stresses the importance of starting by considering how health is created and maintained rather than focusing on the negative aspects of illness and disorder. The salutogenic theory is called the 'break down continuum' (Antonovsky 1972). 'Health ease' is the optimal end of the continuum, while 'dis-ease' is at the opposite end. According to the salutogenic approach, people have access to various resources that can help them to perceive the world as an organised and structured reality. Antonovsky proposed that life experiences produce 'generalised resistance resources', which are positive ways of responding and adapting to new situations.

The SOC theory is firmly located in the person's own context and culture (Antonovsky 1987a, b, 1993). Antonovsky suggested that all humans with or without an illness can experience health and the SOC could be seen as the determinant of the individual's health. In contrast, properties that Antonovsky (1993) called 'generalised resistance deficits' such as low social class, cultural instability and isolation lead to weak SOC. The balance of experiences provided by general resistance resources and generalised resistance deficits in a person's life leads them to a particular location on the SOC continuum (Antonovsky 1992).

Concepts that help balance the resources and deficits in a person's life are:

- Comprehensibility
- Manageability
- Meaningfulness (Antonovsky 1992).

The higher the SOC, the better the person's skills at maintaining and improving their health potential; therefore SOC can be considered to be an internally based coping resource. It determines how a person perceives their environment, for example, stress-free, disturbing or chaotic. External demands such as diabetes self-care should be interpreted as challenges (Antonovsky 1987a, b, p. 135). As people with diabetes grow older the disease, treatment and self-care burdens often increase, which requires a higher level of SOC.

People with a high SOC are aware of their feelings and are capable of controlling their environment and adopting more appropriate behaviour compared to people with a low SOC. People with a low SOC are unsure of their capabilities and are more likely to feel overwhelmed and exposed to an uncontrollable environment (Antonovsky 1987a, b), for example, when moving from home into an aged care facility. Social support is fundamental transitions to living in an aged care home in order to sustain a high SOC.

The construct of SOC is explained as an individual's capacity to respond to stressful situations. The stress is experienced when the outside world impinges on the person's boundaries. The stronger the SOC, the more the person will try to clarify the nature of the particular stressor they are confronting, select resources they believe will be appropriate in the specific situation, and be open to feedback that helps them modify their behaviour. The extent to which a person perceives they understand the situation, have the resources to cope well, and believe it is worth-while to invest effort to manage the challenge affects how the individual responds to stressful situations (Antonovsky 1992).

Older people with diabetes might find it difficult to manage their diabetes during transitions, for example, into widowhood or out of the work workforce. They might not have the resources to cope with the new situation or not believe it is worthwhile to invest the effort; hence thy might regard diabetes management might as a lower priority in their life at that time, which can affect their coping strategies.

The meaningfulness component in SOC theory represents the motivational com-ponent and determines whether a situation is appraised as challenging and whether it is worth making commitments and investments in order to cope (Antonovsky 1987a, b). In order to be motivated to engage in health-creating processes, people need to make sense of events in an emotional as well as a cognitive way. According to Cowley and Billings (1999) 'making sense' involves a person putting symptoms, experiences, treatments, and coping mechanisms in the context of their own family, friends, personal contacts, and reasons for living. The choice of coping mechanisms depends on the factors just described. Older people with diabetes can become over-whelmed to manage life changes and their diabetes concurrently. Social and psy-chological support are vital to encourage older people to manage diabetes and it is meaningful to them; hence the support must be provided on their terms and in their contexts.

7.2   Transitions in Older People

Koelen et al. (2017) said that old age is an accumulation of losses forcing older people to adapt and adjust to constantly changing physical and social environments (Koelen et al. 2017). Antonovsky considered ageing to be a process of human devel-opment instead of just a biological and mental degradation of the body (Antonovsky 1993). He positioned ageing in the context of a health continuum, the ease/disease continuum, and argued that people are all constantly moving in the continuum. People, depending on their age and health status, are in different positions on the health continuum throughout life (Antonovsky 1993).

Most older people demonstrate great ability to find a range of different strategies to deal with these changes. Over time, however, the available options become fewer as a result of declining resources and ability, which can have an impact on the older person's mental health and increase the risk of social isolation, loneliness and depression (Dykstra 2009).

The availability of social contacts and the ability to engage in social interaction are, therefore, important for maintaining healthy ageing and alleviating loneliness. To adapt to changing circumstances, older people may use a range of strategies and tools to engage with their environment, for example, using the Internet through social media, email and Skype which has a significant positive effect on mental well-being of older people (Forsman and Nordmyr 2015) (see Chapter XX).

Using new strategies to manage life transitions aligns with the SOC concept in that recent research indicates that SOC develops over the full life span and in fact increases with age (Feldt et al. 2007, 2011; Nilson et al. 2010). A higher level of SOC increases the old person's ability to cope with everyday life, establish social support, maintain their level of self-confidence and leads to lower mortality rates and less functional decline in individuals with multiple chronic diseases aged 80 and older (Boeckxstaens et al. 2016).

Social connections enrich life for all age groups; however, when people become older, social connections become more and more important (Oswald and Wahl 2005; Puts et al. 2007; Tan et al. 2013). Having responsibility for day-to-day events such as watering plants or looking after a dog enhances psychological well-being, health and activity patterns compared to people with no responsibilities (Puts et al. 2007).

Over the past decade the concept of 'age-friendly communities' emerged. Menec et al. (2011) conceptualised age-friendly communities as shown in Fig. 7.1 (Koelen et al. 2017).

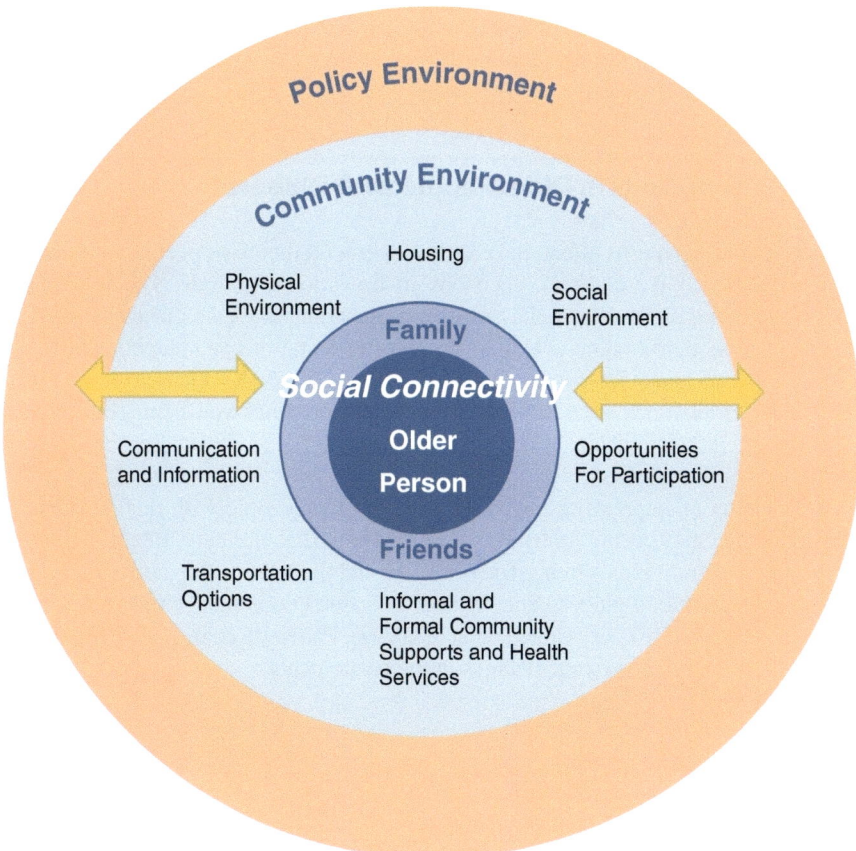

Fig. 7.1 Conceptualising age-friendly communities (Menec et al. 2011, p. 484)

Age-friendly communities create connections between older people and the environment in which they live and vice versa (Menec et al. 2011, p. 484). Thus age-friendly environments, like connectedness very much relate to the SOC dimension of meaningfulness.

Having a purpose in life is closely related to the maintenance of social relationships and increases the likelihood the person will be physically and socially active (Takkinen and Ruoppila 2001). Social connectivity, which is defined as the measure of how people come together and interact, enables older people to recognise and use their internal resources to strengthen one or more of the three dimensions of SOC—meaningfulness, manageability and comprehensibility—which in turn enables them to recognise and use their external resources as needed in specific encounters with stressors (Koelen et al. 2017).

In Australia, the awareness about social connectivity and health is increasing (Pate 2014; ACSA 2015). Many aged care organisations and local councils offer social programmes designed to help older people stay connected to others (COTA 2016). Connectivity can be both formal and informal. It can occur through interaction with family and friends, and planned or spontaneous engagement in the community (Buys et al. 2015), for example, by participation in arts programmes, local community fairs, children 'adopting a grant parent' and child care facilities and schools connected to aged care facilities.

7.3   Transitions in Older People with Diabetes

Changes in life patterns affect diabetes management; therefore people with diabetes often need to make complex decisions in transitional periods. The relationship between managing psychosocial stress and managing diabetes makes people with diabetes particularly vulnerable to a variety of expectations and reactions from others, including health professionals (Kralik et al. 2006; Rasmussen et al. 2007). Successful transitions are described in terms of emotional well-being, mastery and well-being in relationships (Kail and Cavanuagh 2018; Rasmussen et al. 2007; Schumacher and Meleis 1994).

The focus on supporting processes to help older people with diabetes achieve positive outcomes during transitions is pertinent to diabetes care. Research into the experience of individuals living with diabetes and the relationship between the transition process, blood glucose control and the valued outcomes intensified sense of self, meaning and mastery (Paterson et al. 1999). Patterson et al. (1999) found transitions resulted in significant changes in the participants':

- Values
- Health beliefs
- Assumptions and/or
- Daily activities in living with diabetes.

During the transition process the individual learns to restructure the self and the illness experience through the differentiation of the self. This means that the transition process enables individuals to articulate a conscious decision to identify and interpret the challenge and in doing so, create a new relationship with the illness, their social network and with those who provide health care (Paterson et al. 1999). Health professionals (HP) can, therefore, make a unique contribution to assist individuals to achieve a sense of self, empowerment and well-being by being present in encounters, actively listening and asking the 'right' questions and valuing their personal stories, values, beliefs and preferences.

During transitions people might question their identity and sense of self, which results in high levels of uncertainty and difficulty making decisions, emotional instability and withdrawal from social engagements (Heggdal and Lovaas 2017; von Humboldt et al. 2015). Health professionals can empower and preserve older people's sense of self by engaging them in their treatment, developing their abilities to manage their health, helping them express their concerns and preferences regarding treatment and care, encouraging them to ask questions about treatment options, and building strategic patient-provider partnerships through shared decision-making (Chen et al. 2016) (see Chap. 2).

The importance of understanding the physical and pathophysiologic aspects of living with diabetes is imperative for HPs involved in the treatment and care of older people with diabetes. It is often the physical aspects of diabetes, especially diabetes complications or fear thereof, that bring people in contact with health professionals and services in a variety of health care settings.

General care considerations for older people with diabetes aged 75 and older living in aged care facilities relate to their life transition at any time and the processes they use to negotiate the transitions. In addition, the following issues are important.

- Regular general practice reviews, specialist support for complex illnesses, and providing end-of-life diabetes care.
- Diabetes doubles the dementia rate and leads to dependency and compromised self-management skills such as making decisions and administering insulin.
- Frailty is associated with diabetes, ~25% of patients are defined as frail and are at higher risk of falling, becoming functionally impaired, or being hospitalised within the next 12 months.
- Dementia and frailty increase the risk of disabling hypoglycaemia in older people with diabetes treated with sulfonylurea or insulin, the latter accounts for one-fifth of all hospital admissions of older patients with diabetes.
- A quarter of all care home residents have diabetes and they have high rates of infections, foot ulceration and admission into hospital.
- Diabetes education for family and carers is paramount.
- Staff education, including insulin treatment, diabetes care policies, and individualised-care planning, are essential (Sinclair in Hattersley et al. 2014; Dunning et al. 2014a, b).

These factors in mind, combined with the transition theories presented at the beginning of the chapter, suggest that, considering the concepts of activity and participation are essential for older people's well-being during transitions. It is worth noting that von Humboldt et al. (2015) examined the role of SOC and sociodemographic, lifestyle and health-related factors in predicting subjective well-being.

Interestingly, von Humboldt et al. (2015) found that self-reported *spirituality* was the strongest predictor of subjective well-being in older people. Other predictors were sense of coherence, social support, living setting, household, perceived health and medication. Health professionals should be aware of the growing literature indicating a shift in older individuals' sense of well-being when changes occur in regards to their:

- Sense of purpose
- Emotional stability
- Conscious ageing in later life with a possible impact in activity participation
- Social values
- Health care needs (Von Humboldt et al. 2015)

The next section describes some strategies HPs can use to support older during life transitions.

7.4   Role of Health Professionals and Strategies They Can Use to Support Older People with Diabetes During Transitions

Changes in circumstances over time mean people's medical and educational needs change dramatically in older age. Major aims of diabetes care include maintaining independence, functional status and quality of life by reducing symptom and medicine burden and actively identifying risks (Sinclair et al. 2015). It is essential for HPs to assist people through transitions by appropriate care, education, and providing health services based on a personalised care model. Importantly, HPs should avoid ageist stereotypical language, which is disempowering and reduces the individual's personal dignity (Chap. 3).

With the sense of coherence as an underpinning construct, health professionals can identify older people at risk of poor health or reduced quality of life by offering early targeted assistance to strengthen old people's internal and external resources to limit functional decline and enhance their SOC. This can be provided by:

- Promoting active ageing in the community in which the person lives, e.g. stay in their own home as long as possible to maintain their personal dignity independence, sense of security, participation in community activities, pride, familiarity and maintaining relationships with the family and other social networks, freedom, feeling of privacy.
- Identifying available resources and support and helping people adopt coping strategies to empower them to regain a sense of control over their daily activities, e.g. by initiating SOC screening early to identify weak SOC as soon as possible, provide mental health enhancement programmes, positive appraisal and a safe environment.

- Residents in aged care facilities can be helped to mobilise their resources to cope with daily life challenges and experience meaning in the process. For example, HPs can adopt a collaborative and inclusive approach to care and:
  - Provide physical activities for the older person because they enhance well-being and SOC
  - Help them engage with supportive relationships such as family members
  - Encourage personal control
  - Provide safe care through proactive risk assessment and management by understanding the ageing process and impact on the physiological, mental and social health
  - Support them to maintain dignity (Tan et al. 2013; Koelen et al. 2017).

Caring for older adults with diabetes encompasses the need to regularly check older people with diabetes' care plans and goals to accommodate changing circumstances that might involve admission to an aged care home, which often:

- Engenders emotional responses such as grief and distress
- limits functionality
- assists in the transition to palliative care or end-of-life care.

The transition moving from home to an aged care facility is prominent in many older peoples' minds due to the major impact the transition can have on their general well-being, their family and social connectivity as well as their mortality; hence HPs must be knowledgeable about this transition so they can support and collaborate with the older person and their families to achieve a positive transition.

7.5   Transition to Aged Care Facilities

HPs have an integral role assisting older people to make a healthy transition to and successfully adapt to the care home environment. As already stated, the transition is often associated with uncertainty and stress, regardless of whether the transition is welcomed (Bridges 1980). Nurse-patient relationships are often built during transitions that involve developmental, situational or health status changes (Schumacher and Meleis 1994). To be effective in helping older people negotiate transitions HPs need a comprehensive model from which to develop personalised interventions.

Brandburg's (2007) framework is specifically applicable to the transition to aged care homes. It comprises four components:

- Initial reaction
- Transitional influences
- Adjustment
- Acceptance, which can be either adaptive or maladaptive

Initial Reaction: marked by emotional responses such as feeling overwhelmed, disorganised and a sense of homelessness.

Transitional influences and Adjustment: The second and third stages, transitional influences and adjustment, interact in a back-and-forth pattern. There is interplay between these stages during the process of transition, in that older people are in a dynamic process of adjusting and readjusting as they interact with various transitional influences (Brandburg, p. 54). For example, new relationships formed in the aged care home may help older people develop a more positive person-environment network, maintain old friendships and help them reflect on their new home environment. In the SOC construct this would equate to making sense and finding meaning in the transition.

Acceptance: The transition period appears to end when new residents accept living in the care home, which usually occurs between 6 and 12 months after admission (Brooke 1989; Chenitz 1983; Wilson 1997). Descriptions of this period include settling in (Brooke 1989), getting used to it (Porter and Clinton 1992) and acceptance (Wilson 1997).

Acceptance is the outcome of the transitional process and can be adaptive or maladaptive. With adaptive acceptance, older people find meaning in life in the aged care home (Wilson 1997). Maladaptive acceptance can lead to depression, withdrawal and helplessness (Chenitz 1983; Porter and Clinton 1992), which is also described in the SOC construct related to disease versus a salugenetic outcome. Figure 7.2 provides an overview of the Transition Process Framework (REF).

Transitioning into an aged care home can be very challenging. It is important to recognise and acknowledge the multiple changes the older person and their family/carer experience. Often the older person will have experienced a significant decline in their physical health, which is also associated with loss of independence. The move to communal living and a change to every day routines can be very confronting. Similarly, the loss or dispersal of significant objects and belongings, including beloved pets, change in the person's sense of control and sense of place can result in relocation distress syndrome (Walker et al. 2007).

A number of strategies can support people to adjust and make the transition to life in an aged care home, including:

- Effective communication that enables care home staff to get to know the older person (Fraher and Coffey 2011).
- Establishing friendships with other residents and encouraging the individual to engage in recreational and social activities (Fessman and Lester 2000).
- Demonstrating respect and ensuring dignity (Chochinov et al. 2012; Williams et al. 2003).
- Maintaining autonomy by discussing options with the individual and allowing them to make choices (Hollman 2008; Phillipe and Vallerand 2008).
- Empowering the individual by ensuring they are engaged in making choices over as many things as possible (Oosterveld-Vlug et al. 2013)

It is important to remember that HPs' behaviour and attitudes towards older people can have a positive or negative impact on their sense of dignity, self-worth and

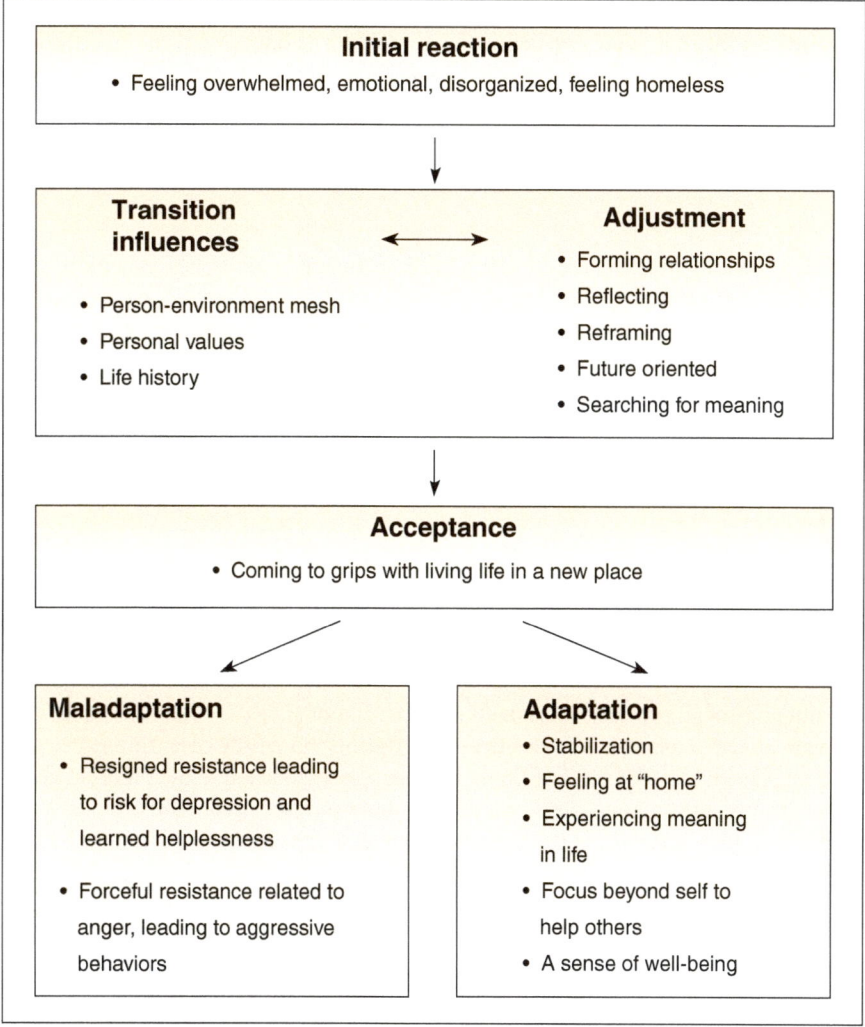

Fig. 7.2 Transition process framework (Brandburg, 2007, p. 54)

place in society (Brandburg et al. 2013). Understanding how best to use these strategies will help HPs have a positive impact when they work with older people; however in terms of specific support during the transition process. Brandburg et al. (2013, p. 187) suggest using the following strategies when caring for people undergoing transitions:

- Assess for positive coping patterns.
- Recognise the individual's ability to deal with past challenges as a way to recognise their strengths.
- Build on past successes to empower the individual to cope with current challenges.

- Help the individual identify the areas he or she can control.
- Support the individual engage in active problem-solving.
- Assist the individual let go of what he or she cannot control.
- Support the individual to build relationships.
- Provide opportunities for the individual to express spirituality.
- Support the individual's expression of hope for the future (Brandburg 2007, p. 187).

HPs working in aged care facilities need to engage in numerous transitions older people make; ultimately they frequently work with older people in the transition to their end of life. HPs have an important role in easing, managing and negotiating the transition to end-of-life care (Brandburg 2007). Ideally, end-of-life care planning should occur in a supportive environment and include all relevant people when discussing older people's people's goals, values and preferences and documenting advance care plans. Ideally advance care planning and documenting and advanced care directive should occur before the older person is admitted to an aged care home.

7.6   End-of-Life Transitions

For many people, the last few months of life involve the most intensive contact with health and social services (Forma et al. 2009; Pot et al. 2009). HP face many challenges and need to make complex decisions during end-of-life care. Life expectancy has increased; therefore end of life is increasingly associated with comorbid conditions, frailty and smaller family units to provide support (Lynn 2005; Seale 2005). Adding to these changes is the transition between services such as from one health service to home or vice versa.

Hanratty et al. (2012) undertook a qualitative study in palliative care and found that, as older people moved between different settings, much of the care they received was characterised by inflexibility, liaison between and within services was not always effective, and community support after a hospital admission was perceived as inadequate. However, Hanratty et al. suggest that HPs are able to facilitate good clinical practice at the end of life of older people when:

- Communication between individuals and HPs is respectful.
- Coordination takes place across services that recognise individuals' need and wishes.
- There is planned transfer of responsibility to family doctors, carers and/or social care when relevant.
- HP treat the whole person and listen to them.
- Dignity is upheld (Hanratty et al. 2012)

These practice strategies are reflected in both Dunning et al.'s (2010) *Guidelines for Managing Diabetes at the End of Life* report and Dunning et al.'s (2014a, b)

McKellar Guidelines for Managing Older People with Diabetes in Residential and Other Care Settings. Dunning et al. provide extensive guidelines for end-of-life care. The following strategies reflect end-of-life care transitions:

- *Monitor the individual's general and diabetes health status* to identify clinical deterioration early and implement diabetes-specific management strategies, which might be to implement palliative care and the person's end-of-life care plan and advance care directive.
- *Consider whether the individual would benefit from referral for supportive care/ palliative approach* according to their end-of-life stage. Supportive care can be commenced at any time not just at the end of life.
- *Religious and spiritual support* should be offered to the individual and their family.
- Determine whether individual has an Advance Care Directive (ACD) in place. If not, discuss the issues with the individual and/or their family and document an ACD and/or other proxy decision-making information. Note: The legislation and regulations concerning advanced care planning and other related end-of-life issues vary among countries, and often states within countries.

HPs need to assess and meet the needs of the dying person and their family, provide good communication based on the suggested strategies, and respect the person's dignity and attend to their spiritual and/or religious wishes/needs when they engage with older people with diabetes in their end-of-life transition.

7.7 Chapter Summary

HPs need to carefully examine the old persons' experiences to fully understand the strategies they use to manage diabetes and transition-related changes at the same time. HPs need to be aware that previous diabetes management strategies are inadequate in changing environments and new coping strategies are needed. The transition process may also trigger a shift in perceptions of how to manage diabetes.

Thus, when interacting with older people with diabetes HPs need to acknowledge the shift and collaborate with the older person and their families to optimise their diabetes management and reduce the impact of complications. Health professionals need to negotiate 'with' older adults not 'for' them, and develop management plans that reflect older people's altered life values and perceptions.

7.8 Reflective Questions

Life transitions are commonly spoken about in our day-to-day lives because everyone experiences special events, which might become turning points in their lives. Often more than one transition occurs at once which adds challenges for everyone involved in the person's care. This chapter presented different transition theories and indicated the role of health professionals in implementing strategies to support older people during transition(s). The following questions might help you to reflect on what you have just read.

- Thinking back on your own life, can you recall a transition or two that changed your life or outlook on life (attitudes, motivation)?
- Which emotions do your recall from that period in your life?
- Think about which strategies helped you through the transition(s)?
- Which obstacles did you encounter, and how did you negotiate them?
- Are the strategies you used to manage transitions applicable to your practice?
- Are they applicable older people with diabetes?
- What was the most useful information in this chapter?

References

Aged and Community Service Australia (ACSA) (2015) *A issues paper: social isolation and loneliness*—October 2015

Antonovsky A (1972) Breakdown: a needed fourth step in the conceptual armamentarium of modern medicine. Soc Sci Med 6:537–544

Antonovsky A (1979) Health, stress and coping. Jossey-Bass Publishers, San Francisco

Antonovsky A (1987a) Unraveling the mystery of health—how people manage stress and stay well. Jossey-Bass Publishers, San Francisco

Antonovsky A (1987b) Unravelling the mystery of health. Jossey-Bass Inc., San Francisco

Antonovsky A (1992) Can attitudes contribute to health? ADVANCES. J Mind-Body Health 8(4):33–49

Antonovsky A (1993) The structure and properties of the sense of coherence scale. Soc Sci Med 36:725–733

Boeckxstaens P, Vaes B, De Sutter A, Aujoulat I, van Pottelbergh G, Matheï C, Degryse J (2016) A high sense of coherence as protection against adverse health outcomes in patients aged 80 years and older. Ann Fam Med 14(4):337–343

Brandburg GL (2007) Making the transition to nursing home life: a framework to help older adults adapt to the long-term care environment. J Gerontol Nurs 33(6):50–56

Brandburg GL, Symes L, Mastel-Smith B, Hersch G, Walsh T (2013) Resident strategies for making a life in a nursing home: a qualitative study. J Adv Nurs 69(4):862–874. https://doi.org/10.1111/j.1365-2648.2012.06075.x

Bridges W (2001) Transitions: making sense of life's changes. Nicholas Brealey Publishing, London

Bridges W (2002) Managing transitions: making the most of change. Nicholas Brealey Publishing, London

Brooke V (1989) How elders adjust. Geriatr Nurs 10:66–68

Buys L, Burton L, Cuthill M, Hogan A, Wilson B, Baker D (2015) Establishing and maintaining social connectivity: an understanding of the lived experiences of older adults residing in regional and rural communities. Aust J Rural Health 23(5):291–294

Chen J et al (2016) Personalized strategies to activate and empower patients in health care and reduce health disparities. Health Educ Behav 43(1):25–34

Chenitz WC (1983) Entry into a nursing home as status passage: a theory to guide nursing practice. Geriatr Nurs 4:92–97

Chochinov HM, Cann B, Cullihall K, Kristjanson L, Harlos M, McClement SE (2012) Dignity therapy: a feasibility study of elders in long term care. Palliat Support Care 10(1):3–15

COTA (2016) For older Australians. http://www.cota.org.au/australia/aboutus/strategic-directions-2016-2020.aspx. Accessed 7 Oct 2017

Cowley S, Billings JR (1999) Resources revisited: salutogenesis from a lay perspective. J Adv Nurs 29(4):994–1004

Dunning T, Martin P, Savage S, Duggan N (2010) Guidelines for managing diabetes at the end of life report. Centre for Nursing and Allied Health, Deakin University, Geelong

Dunning T, Sinclair A, Colagiuri S (2014a) New IDF guideline for managing type 2 diabetes in older people. Diabetes Res Clin Pract 103(3):538–540

Dunning T, Duggan N, Savage S (2014b) The McKellar guidelines for managing older people with diabetes in residential and other care settings. Centre for Nursing and Allied Health, Deakin University, Geelong

Dykstra PA (2009) Older adult loneliness: myths and realities. Eur J Ageing 6:91–100

Feldt T, Lintula H, Suominen S, Koskenvuo M, Vahtera J, Kivimäki M (2007) Structural validity and temporal stability of the 13-item sense of coherence scale: prospective evidence from the population-based HeSSup study. Qual Life Res 16:483–493

Feldt T, Leskinen E, Koskenvuo M, Suominen S, Vahtera J, Kivimäki M (2011) Development of sense of coherence in adulthood: a person-centered approach. The population-based HeSSup cohort study. Qual Life Res 20:69–79

Fessman N, Lester D (2000) Loneliness and depression among elderly nursing home patients. Int J Aging Hum Dev 51(2):137–141

Forma L, Rissanen P, Aaltonen M, Raitanen J, Jylha M (2009) Age and closeness of death as determinants of health and social care utilization: a case-control study. Eur J Public Health 19:313–318

Forsman AK, Nordmyr J (2015) Psychosocial links between Internet use and mental health in later life: a systematic review of quantitative and qualitative evidence. J Appl Gerontol:1–48. https://doi.org/10.1177/07334648155955096

Fraher A, Coffey A (2011) Older people's experiences of relocation to long-term care. Nurs Older People 23(10):23–27

Hanratty B et al (2012) Older adults' experiences of transitions between care settings at the end of life in England: a qualitative interview study. J Pain Symptom Manage 44(1):74–83

Hattersley AT, Marcovecchio ML, Chiarelli F, Silverstein J, Heller S, Damm P, Mathiesen ER, Zinmann B, Sinclair A (2014) Lifecourse: management of type 1 diabetes. Lancet Diabetes Endocrinol 2(3):194–195. https://doi.org/10.1016/S2213-8587(13)70179-7

Heggdal K, Lovaas BJ (2017) Health promotion in specialist and community care: how a broadly applicable health promotion intervention influences patient's sense of coherence. Scand J Caring Sci (not fully published yet)

Hollman C (2008) Living bereavement: An exploration of healthcare workers responses to loss and grief in an NHS continuing care ward for older people. Int J Older People Nurs 3(4):278–281

von Humboldt S, Leal I, Pimenta F (2015) Sense of coherence, sociodemographic, lifestyle, and health-related factors in older adults' subjective well-being. Int J Gerontol 9(1):15–19

Kail RV, Cavanuagh JC (2018) Human development: a life-span view, 8 eds. Cengage Learning, Boston

Koelen M, Eriksson M, Cattan M (2017) Older people, sense of coherence and community. In: Mittelmark MB, Sagy S, Eriksson M et al (eds) The handbook of salutogenesis. Springer International Publishing, Cham, pp 137–149

Kralik D, van Loon A (2007) Understanding transition in chronic illness. Aust Nurs J 15(2):29–35

Kralik D, Visentin K, van Loon A (2006) Transition: a literature review. J Adv Nurs 55:320–329. https://doi.org/10.1111/j.1365-2648.2006.03899.x. Accessed 23 Jul 2017

Lynn J. (2005) Living long in fragile health: the new demographics shape end of life care. Hastings Cent Rep S14eS18. Spec No

Menec VH, Means R, Jeating N, Parkhurst G, Eales J (2011) Conceptualizing age-friendly communities. Can J Aging 30(3):479–493

Nilsson K, Leppert J, Simonsson B, Starrin B (2010) Sense of coherence (SOC) and psychological well-being (GHQ): improvement with age. J Epidemiol Community Health 64(4):347–352

Oosterveld-Vlug MG, Pasman HRW, van Gennip IE, Muller MT, Willems DL (2013) Dignity and factors that influence it according to nursing home residents: a qualitative study. J Adv Nurs 70(1):97–106

Oswald F, Wahl HW (2005) Dimensions of the meaning of home in later life. In: Rowles GD, Chaudhury H (eds) Home and identity in late life: international perspectives. Springer, New York, pp 21–45

Pate A (2014) Social isolation: its impact on the mental health of older Victorians', *COTA Victoria,* Working Paper No. 1, 6

Paterson BL et al (1998) Adapting to and managing diabetes. Image J Nurs Sch 30(1):57–62

Paterson BL, Thorne SE, Crawford J, Tarko M (1999) Living with diabetes as a transformational experience. Qual Health Res 9(6):786–803

Phillipe F, Vallerand R (2008) Actual environments do affect motivation and psychological adjustment: a test of self-determination theory in a natural setting. Motiv Emot 32(2):81–89

Polonsky WH, Fisher L, Earles J, Dudl RJ, Lees J, Mullan J, Jackson RA (2005) Assessing psychosocial distress in diabetes development of the diabetes distress scale. Diabetes Care 28:626–631. https://doi.org/10.2337/diacare.28.3.626. Accessed 23 Jul 2017

Porter EJ, Clinton JF (1992) Adjusting to the nursing home. West J Nurs Res 14:464–481

Pot AM, Portrait F, Visser G, Puts M, Broese van Groenou MI, Deeg DJH (2009) Utilization of acute and long-term care in the last year of life: comparison with survivors in a population-based study. BMC Health Serv Res 9:139

Puts MTE, Shekary N, Widdershoven G, Helders PJ, Lips P, Deeg DJH (2007) What does quality of life mean to older frail and non-frail community-dwelling adults in the Netherlands? Qual Life Res 16:263–277

Rasmussen B, O'Connell B, Dunning T, Cox H (2007) Young women with type 1 diabetes: management of turning points and transitions. Qual Health Res 17:300–310. https://doi.org/10.1177/1049732306298631. Accessed 23 Jul 2017

Schlossberg NK et al (1995) Counseling adults in transition linking practice with theory. Springer, New York

Schumacher KL, Meleis AI (1994) Transitions: a central concept in nursing. Image J Nurs Sch 26:119–127

Seale C (2005) Changing patterns of death and dying. Soc Sci Med 51:917–930

Sinclair A, Dunning T, Rodriguez-Mañas L (2015) Diabetes in older people: new insights and remaining challenges. Lancet Diabetes Endocrinol 3:275–285

Takkinen S, Ruoppila I (2001) Meaning in life in three samples of elderly persons with high cognitive functioning. Int J Aging Hum Dev 53(1):51–73

Tan K-K, Vehviläinen-Julkunen K, Chan SW (2013) Integrative review: salutogenesis and health in older people over 65 years old. J Adv Nurs 70(3):497–510

Walker CA, Curry LC, Hogstel MO (2007) Relocation stress syndrome in older adults transitioning from home to long term care facility. Myth or reality? J Psychosoc Nurs Ment Health Serv 45(1):38–45

Williams K, Kemper S, Hummert ML (2003) Improving nursing home communication: an intervention to reduce elderspeak. Gerontologist 43(2):242–247

Wilson SA (1997) The transition to nursing home life: a comparison of planned and unplanned admissions. J Adv Nurs 26:864–871

Personalising Care with Older People Who Have Cognitive Changes or Dementia

8

Kirsten James and Trisha Dunning

I am daily learning to be the reluctant guardian of your memories. There was light in those eyes; I miss that.

(Ratliff R)

Key Points

- Impaired cognition is complex; it can be temporary, degenerative and static and/ or fluctuate. Considered, collateral, individualised assessments, accurate diagnosis and regular reviews in consultation with the person and their carers are vital to help to determine appropriate personalised management and care.
- An older person's life story, including past social and medical history are as important as their current circumstances. They provide context for their plan of care and personalised treatment. Capturing this information can help carers to focus on the person's strengths and support their wishes.
- Impaired cognition does not replace an individual's right to self-determination or prevent them from expressing their preferences and participating in care decisions. Situations can be fraught as cognition declines or is acutely compromised. Importantly, the contribution carers make and the significant care work professional and family carers undertake should never be taken for granted.
- Proactive engagement with older people and their carers in the early stages of cognitive decline as well as during 'windows of clarity and lucidity' are the 'right times' to plan, document and share information. The principles of dignity

K. James, M.H.Sci. Grad. Dip. Ad. Ed. & Tg (✉)
Cohealth, Melbourne, VIC, Australia
e-mail: Kirsten.James@cohealth.org.au

T. Dunning, A.M., M.Ed., Ph.D., R.N., C.D.E.
Centre for Quality and Patient Safety Research, Barwon Health Partnership,
Deakin University, Geelong, VIC, Australia
e-mail: trisha.dunning@barwonhealth.org.au;
trisha.dunning@deakin.edu.au

© Springer International Publishing AG, part of Springer Nature 2018
T. Dunning (ed.), *The Art and Science of Personalising Care with Older People with Diabetes*, https://doi.org/10.1007/978-3-319-74360-8_8

and respect can be used to guide and support older people, their carers and health professionals to make choices, promote independence and minimise risk.

- Care needs to be goal-directed, holistic, personalised, realistic, and adaptable to accommodate changing circumstances. Sometimes carers have to change their expectations. Lateral thinking and creative, practical strategies can help address problems and decide effective outcomes.

8.1   Introduction

Dementia is a global challenge associated with longevity and affects 47 million people globally, most are age 65 and older (Lancet Commission 2017). Risk factors for dementia include the following risk factors, some of which could be reduced by a healthy lifestyle and social connections:

- Genetic predisposition
- Social isolation
- Hearing loss
- Inadequate exercise
- Inappropriate diet
- Smoking
- Depression and other mental health disorders
- Diabetes, which is associated with all types of dementia including vascular, Alzheimer's and Lewy bodies.
- Hypertension
- Mild cognitive impairment (Lancet Commission 2017).

All major mental health disorders are associated with effects on cognitive performance (Geerlings et al. 2000; Rock et al. 2013) and people presenting to a memory or dementia clinic have a 40–50% chance of developing a mental health condition (Fisher 2017). Mental health disorders and dementia affect executive functions including memory, processing speed, language and alertness. Therefore, screening for mental health conditions and asking about drug and alcohol use is important. Cognitive enrichment programmes that support positive attitudes and social engagement influence health behaviours (Hertzog et al. 2009) and may be important risk minimise strategies.

Age is the greatest risk factor for cognitive impairment, and as the Baby Boomer population, those born between post World War 2 and 1964, reach age 65, the number of people living with dementia is expected to jump dramatically (Alzheimer's Disease International 2013). The United Nations (UN) (2015) indicated the number of older people tripled in the last 50 years and will triple again over the next 50 years. Although developed regions have relatively high proportions of older people, there is a faster growth rate of older people in less developed regions (UN 2015; World Health Organisation (WHO 2015).

This situation will create overwhelming demands on global communities and health systems. An estimated >20% of the global population will be older than 65 by 2050 and there will be fewer people to take care of them (Gill 2015, UN 2015). In addition, there is a corresponding decline in the number of specialists training in geriatric medicine, which will create other care challenges for health professionals (HP), service providers and society (Girdwain 2011; RACP and ANZSGM 2012; Hafner 2016) and may affect safety and the quality of care.

Cognitive changes can occur during hypoglycaemia and hyperglycaemia or be a long-term complication of diabetes and other factors. Many health professionals, family carers and people with diabetes incorrectly believe people cannot be engaged in care decisions if they are cognitively impaired. This chapter will encompass "the right time and right way" to discuss care with older people and cognitive impairment. The role of lateral problem-solving and other creative ways to care will be considered.

8.2   Overview of Changes in the Brain as People Get Older

Changes that occur in the brain are part of general 'slowing down'. Fear of dementia is a major concern for most older people and their families. Biologically, brain ageing begins early, even from the twenties. There is a small but continuous loss of white matter, which means the number of myelinated axons that carry fast information around the brain are decreasing. The brain is adept at compensating for changes and build new connections.

Cellular research shows brain plasticity continues in the eighties and older people generally become more knowledgeable and practiced at doing things; their vocabulary increases and they can generally problem-solve except under time pressure.

- Some parts of the brain are particularly vulnerable to the effects of ageing, e.g. the limbic system and the prefrontal cortex.
- Older people may become a little less inhibited and take less time to think before making decisions. Encouraging them to reflect on important issues might avoid inappropriate decisions.
- Some older people become 'set in their ways'.
- Memory lapses increase in frequency with older age. However, some mental abilities improve with age. Some people are resilient to the effects of age. They often find it difficult to remember things that have no specific relevance to them. Cues to memory, giving people more time to think and do things, and avoiding distractions help.
- A healthy diet, regular exercise, adequate sleep and continuing to use the brain are important protective activities. They are also key diabetes management strategies and help maintain cardiovascular health.
- Cardiovascular health is essential to carry oxygen and nutrient to the brain and remove waste products and toxins.
- Cognitive functions most commonly affected by age are:
  - thinking speed—ability to make quick decisions, process directions, mental arithmetic

- executive functions such as planning ahead, using complex strategies and being flexible such as change of plans
- memory, especially recalling people's names and word finding. (The Curious Minds Series, The Twilight Years in *How it Works: Book of the Brain* future publishing 116–125).

8.3   Diabetes and Dementia

The global prevalence of diabetes is also increasing. Diabetes affects cognition in a number of ways (see Chap. 1). More than 46.8 million people are living with dementia in 2017 and the number is estimated to reach 131.5 million by 2050 (Alzheimer's Disease International (ADI) 2015). Pre-diabetes and diabetes are associated with cognitive impairment, accelerated cognitive decline and contribute to dementia in older adults (Velayudhan et al. 2009, McCrimmon et al. 2012, Biessels et al. 2014; Marseglia et al. 2016). People with diabetes have greater decline in cognitive function and are 1.4-2 times more likely to develop dementia than people without diabetes (Puttanna et al. 2017).

Glycaemic control is associated with declining cognitive function (DCCT/EDIC 2014). The Accord-Mind trial showed that there is a 0.14 drop in the MMSE score for every 1% rise in HbA1c. Glucose variability might also play a role (Chap. 1). Hypoglycaemia also increases the risk of short- and long-term cognitive impairment and can occur at any HbA1c level (Lipska et al. 2013). The symptoms of hypoglycaemia change with duration of diabetes and hypoglycaemia might not be recognised or treated. In the short term important cognitive functions such as problem-solving and decision-making are compromised.

Diabetes and dementia share common lifestyle risk factors. Both are associated with disabling complications, which present considerable management challenges for the person with dementia and diabetes and for their carers and HPs. These challenges include difficulty recognising symptoms of undiagnosed diabetes, hyper- and hypoglycaemia and complications, problem-solving and being able to follow and/or remember lifestyle and medical advice. These factors place the person with diabetes and cognitive impairment at higher risk of under- or overtreatment, adverse events, hospital admission and mortality (McCrimmon et al. 2012; Dunning et al. 2014; Hill 2015).

A number of metabolic, vascular, endocrine and central nervous system factors contribute to the development of cognitive dysfunction in diabetes. For example, chronic or acute hyper- or hypoglycaemia, micro- and macrovascular disease, and depression (McCrimmon et al. 2012). Evidence shows hypertension, obesity and diabetes all impair cognition (The Lancet Commission on Dementia Prevention, Intervention, and Care 2017). However, sensory changes such as sight and hearing can also contribute to disorientation and confusion. It is important that these sensory changes are considered and managed and the person has their glasses and hearing aids checked and maintained, and especially used during care encounters.

Therefore it is important to encourage early diagnosis of both conditions by considering the possibility at every consultation and undertaking targeted screening when indicated. Early diagnosis of both diseases enable baseline and parameters to be collected to guide treatment plans, timely access to support services, manage complications to reduce the associated risk and as a basis for ongoing monitoring (TREND 2013).

Retinal sensitivity is related to cognitive status and the MRI, and 18 FDG-PET parameters related to brain neurodegeneration (Ciudin et al. 2017). Thus, retinal microperimetry may be a new non-invasive way to identify people with diabetes at risk of dementia (Ciudin et al. 2017).

Cognitive impairment can occur in people with T1DM and T2DM and affect motor and mental processing speed, executive functioning and attention. A primary distinguishing feature between T1DM and T2DM is that people with T2DM often demonstrate learning and memory deficits, but these deficits are seen rarely in T1DM. As indicated, diabetes-related effects on cognition can be transient or permanent. Transient changes can be due to high or low blood glucose (McCrimmon et al. 2012).

With more people living longer there will be larger numbers of people experiencing declines in physical and mental capacity who may need care for day-to-day activities…there is a pressing need to develop comprehensive community-based approaches to prevent declines in capacity and to provide support for family caregivers (WHO, ICOP Guidelines 2016).

8.4   Considerations When Deciding Diabetes Management for a Person with Dementia

It is essential to develop practical, flexible care and education plans that individuals and their carers can adapt to suit their changing needs. Planning includes discussing and documenting Advanced Care Directives when the person has capacity to understand the implications of their decisions and make informed decisions. The person's blood glucose at the time, environment in which such discussions occur, the way the information is presented and the time allowed affect the individual's ability to participate in decision-making. It is important not to create cognitive overload.

Key management interventions include:

- Managing metabolic risks: hypertension and hyperglycaemia.
- Providing a rich environment that includes sensory and cognitive stimulation as well as social connections.
- Healthy diet, activity and sleep.
- Using technology to make early diagnosis and keep the individual safe, e.g. wearable sensors, assistive technology and safety devices (see Chap. 9).
- Using reminiscence-based communication, which encompasses:
  - introducing themselves
  - explaining what is happening

- doing one thing at a time and using a step-by-step approach
- avoiding negative language and verbal communication
- allowing the person time to respond
- help them find words

8.5   Impaired Cognition: A Complex Phenomenon

Cognition refers to the mental process involved in knowing, learning and understanding things (Collins 2011). Processes such as thinking, remembering, judging and problem-solving involve high level brain functioning such as imagination, perception, planning and problem-solving. If one or more of these processes are affected cognition can be impaired, depending on the underlying cause. Cognitive impairment can also manifest as acute and temporary, chronic and degenerative, fluctuating and unpredictable. It does not necessarily present as a linear, predictable occurrence but can sometimes seem random and unexpected. In some instances, bystanders may not understand that a person's behaviour change could be due to their medical condition. Consequently appropriate treatment may be delayed or not provided, making the situation worse.

The son had arranged for his older mother to be admitted to an aged care home because she had 'cognitive impairment.'

Aunty Joan, Doc Martin's aunt and the lady's long-time friend visited her every morning to make her a cup of tea. She has cellulitis of one leg, which affected her mobility.

Doc Martin assessed the lady's cognition for orientation to time and place at Aunty Joan's request because the lady did not want to go, and, in Aunty Joan's opinion she was 'not demented.'

She stayed at home. During a subsequent visit, later in the day, the lady was disoriented and refusing to drink because she did not want to be incontinent. She had been limiting her fluid to her morning cup of tea because she could not get to the toilet and was very concerned about 'wetting herself.'

Dehydration was the underlying cause of her confusion/cognitive changes. This anecdote shows there can be physiological causes of or contributors to impaired cognition. These include:

- Delirium, which can be caused by acute infection, severe pain, hyper- and hypo-glycaemia, gastrointestinal disturbances, liver failure and medication side effects.
- Intellectual disability, mental health issues including depression or psychosis, dementia, acquired brain injury (stroke, head injury), alcohol and drug abuse.

Multi-disciplinary teams working together to support the individual and communicate through the primary care provider, often a GP, and supported by a designated personal carer, can make a big difference for the individual with diabetes and cognitive impairment. The author's personal experience suggests some allied health staff are disinclined to report changes in a person's behaviour, yet, with the person or their legal representative's permission, sharing their concerns can be very helpful to alert the GP and to trigger further assessments and earlier access to treatments.

There is some debate about the best screening tools to use to assess cognitive impairment and dementia. In UK, the Mini Cog is used because it is a simple, quick test with 83% accuracy that can indicate whether a person has normal or abnormal cognition (Sinclair et al. 2013). Folstein's Mini-Mental State Examination (MMSE) is widely used to screen for dementia screening. However, it has limitations for people from culturally and linguistically diverse backgrounds and does not assess frontal lobe function, which is involved with executive functions such as problem-solving, impulse control, understanding consequences and socially appropriate behaviour.

The Rowland Universal Dementia Assessment Scale (RUDAS) is increasingly used as an alternative to the MMSE because it effectively discerns deficits and is not affected by culture, language or gender. RUDAS also has high predictive accuracy in a broad population sample for a range of cognitive functions.

The Montreal Cognitive Assessment (MoCA) is also a rapid screening instrument and is useful to detect mild cognitive dysfunction. It assesses multiple cognitive domains and takes approximately 10 min. Regardless of what cognitive screening tool is used it is important that a specialist undertakes a formal comprehensive assessment, for example, in a specialist memory service. The assessment should include a full dementia screen including thyroid function test, serum vitamin B12 and brain scan and electroencephalogram (NICE 2010; TREND UK 2013). Repeated, periodical screening is useful to monitor improvement/decline and to ensure the care plan continues to suit the individual's needs, preferences and goals and consider family carers needs and health.

8.6   Understanding the Impact of Dementia

Diagnosing dementia is a start, but HPs, the individual and family all need to understand the differing impact on all concerned. Ideally, a specialist such as a Neuropsychologist, Geriatrician or Old Age Psychiatrist is consulted to refine the diagnosis, analyse the results of tests and investigations and discuss how to identify and use the individual's strengths to conserve cognitive function, mental and physical health and involve them where possible. For example, a person's memory is not always affected. When memory is, it can be affected in different ways depending on the part/s of the brain involved, the underlying cause of the cognitive impairment, and whether the dementia is in an early or advanced stage.

Understanding the impact of dementia on the person's cognition can help them, their families, friends and other carers find ways to accommodate the changes and select appropriate memory aids and cues to reduce stress demands on all involved.

With appropriate and personalised modifications and visual supports, people with dementia can participate in lifelong interests and hobbies, maintain personal identities and roles in the community, and maintain a quality of life that is noticed and valued by others (Bourgeois et al. 2005).

Examples include:

- Engaging in meaningful, pleasurable and personalised activity programmes that may reconnect the person to skills and experiences from their past work or home life, hobbies and interests.
- Modifying the environment, including the reduction of clutter and ambient noise, ensuring adequate lighting, home-like/familiar furniture and rooms and providing simple, legible instructions as way-finding and instructional cues (The Lancet Commission 2017).
- 'Taking it slow'

This is MY Story: Please do not define me by my illness!

Everybody has a story. When we don't take the time to know someone's story or worse, create our own version of it, we lose the chance to understand what they need which is the first step to empathy. (Acuff 2017)

The traditional medical model of health assessment emphasises the medical history and pays less consideration to the importance of the person's life story. The importance of people's stories, how to elicit them, understand them and use them to plan care with the individual and their families is discussed in Chap. 3. Stories could have another significant role for people with dementia by helping emphasise the individual's personhood and conserve their dignity. They also help HPs have a conversation with an individual and conserve their life history for their families.

Older people are often judged on the basis of their physical appearance. For example, others might consider a thin older person as fragile and vulnerable and miss the frailty in an overweight person. Such judgements arise from ignorance and are perpetuated through stereotypical and ageist attitudes.

Interactions are challenging when the individual has sensory deficits such as hearing or vision impairment. Mobility compromises self-care. Cognitive overload can occur in the 'busy-ness' of hospital, Emergency Department, GP practice and community health clinics and make it difficult for HPs to assess cognitive function. Often they label the person confused and do not try strategies such as speaking clearly, more slowly, using simple sentence structure and avoiding jargon, or using visual prompts to communicate with them. Sometimes family members are consulted for information rather than the person themselves, to save time.

To ignore the person's prior knowledge, life experience, belief systems and preferred ways of learning, as well as their goals and preferences makes it difficult for HPs to truly develop personalised care plans and conserve the individual's dignity, see Chap. 3.

We are teachers and students to each other (Jampolsky 2000)

The individual's living arrangements and circumstances are important aspects of their story and provide context for personalising their treatment and care. An older person with cognitive impairment and diabetes can be compromised by difficult environmental conditions including unstable housing or homelessness, limited income, and either no carer or an inappropriate carer who may subject them to some form of elder abuse including physical and financial abuse. Inadequate health literacy, language difficulties and access to transport can further complicate an individual's access to appropriate, timely care and support. These situations impact food and fluid intake, quality of sleep, access to monitoring equipment and medications, medical and care support and engender significant stress that further compounds the individual's ability to cope and may result in mental health issues including anxiety, depression and suicidal thoughts. Families and HPs should take an older person talking about 'wanting to die' seriously. It is a warning sign that the issue needs to be discussed sensitively and the person referred for treatment and advice (Ganzine in Rapport 2017).

Capturing both the life story and medical history in a practical format to share with relevant service and care providers can be challenging due to issues such as access, privacy and the need to accommodate frequent changes. Life story 'passports' that the cognitively compromised person and/or their carer can take with them to new medical appointments, allied health and respite care providers can be helpful. The other advantage of utilising such records is the individual does not have to rely on memory in stressful new situations and avoids the need to repeat themselves.

'Passports' are also helpful for new residents of nursing homes to share with the staff and help staff 'see the individual as a whole human being'. Many dementia care and support organisations promote the use of story templates that record cultural background, life history, personality, spirituality, values and beliefs, social connections and support networks, sexuality, interests and hobbies, significant life events as well as habits and routines. These can be adapted into different formats, including "Life Story Boxes" and wall displays in the person's bedroom, Life Story DVDs, and Memory wallets and Memory Boards that the person can carry with them (Bourgeois et al. 2005; Alzheimer's Australia Tasmania 2017; Alzheimer's Australia, 2017a, b).

8.7   When the Going Gets Tough...

Most diabetes and cognitive impairment management guidelines do not address some of the most concerning and distressing behaviours that can occur with acute delirium and advanced dementia. Personal and professional carers are often inadequately skilled and trained to respond appropriately in hospital, community and residential care settings (Burns et al. 2012; Sinclair et al. 2014). Unfortunately, the complexity of both conditions in addition to other co-existing comorbidities makes care challenging. Medical training as well as public education and information about both subjects has raised awareness about appropriate assessment and care in recent years, in keeping with the World Health Organization ICOP Guidelines (2016), but there appears to be a lot more work to do.

For example, over 90% of people with dementia will develop Behavioural & Psychological Symptoms of Dementia (BPSDs) at some time during the course of their illness (International Psychogeriatric Association 1996). BPSDs are the noncognitive symptoms of dementia such as disturbed perception, thought, content, mood and behaviour. Examples include physical and verbal aggression, pacing, restlessness and wandering, sleep disturbance, apathy, anxiety, hallucinations, delusions, misidentifications and sexualised behaviours (International Psychogeriatric Association 2002).

According to Sinclair et al. (2015) 'Major aims of diabetes care include maintenance of independence, functional status, and quality of life by reduction of symptom and medicine burden, and active identification of risks'. However, the added diagnosis of dementia can make management challenging for everybody involved in care. For example, the individual can misinterpret blood glucose checks, glucose lowering medicines and giving insulin injections as invasive and threatening. They may react violently (physically and/or verbally) because they do not understand or remember why they are important.

Comprehensive, person-centred assessment is important to:

Prevent. Know the person well—encourage carers to maintain physical and emotional equilibrium through a person-centred approach to engagement/occupation in daily activities; avoid triggers such as boredom, changes in environment and medication. Also, have routine checks with flexible blood glucose level limits to accommodate changes in behaviour.

Minimise. As soon as behaviour change is noticed, prompt assessment to exclude organic causes should be undertaken. If the person is agitated, try again later. Avoid making the situation worse. Address unmet needs before trying other methods such as distraction. Physical exercise and mental stimulation activities can be helpful to induce natural tiredness.

Manage. Prompt critical analysis of pain, behaviour, delirium screening; ask— what is the problem and who is it a problem for? Refer to care plan and ensure that GP has included flexible reportable levels and management strategies. If blood tests are to be required, make it 'count', e.g. undertake multiple pathology tests at the same time. Having blood taken is often distressing for the cognitively impaired person who is not only unlikely to accept, but will probably not understand or remember a rational explanation for taking the blood. Food and fluid charting may be advised during a period of ill-health to ensure adequate intake and to avoid hypo- or hyperglycaemia.

8.7.1 What's Going on with the Carer?

Another consideration is the role and health and well-being of the carer/s: personal and professional. It is important not to presume that:

- The person is cooperative, has a stable carer or number of carers who all get along well with the person and each other.
- That the carer has the person's best interests in mind.
- That the carer understands what is required to care for the person, is coping and is able and willing to seek help if required.

- That the primary care provider can and does review the person on a regular basis and makes appropriate treatment adjustments that are being followed.
- Provides appropriate general health checks and vaccinations when required.
- That all members of the health and care team are qualified and skilled sufficiently to minimise/manage the person's condition, and on the 'same page' and
- Are able and willing to follow a goal-directed care plan that is in line with the person's aims, wishes and is tailored to suit their individual circumstances.

Caring for older people, especially when they have multiple comorbidities like cognitive impairment and diabetes, can be particularly burdensome and stressful. Family and friends can experience higher levels of depression than non-carers, social isolation, disruption to sleep leading to exhaustion, deterioration in physical health, need time off from paid work which can impact on finances, and have feelings of sadness, grief, guilt and persistent worry (Adelman et al. 2014; Alzheimer's Australia 2017a, b).

Lack of control and frustration can sometimes develop into anger and the carer may act out towards the person they are caring for. Others involved may need to monitor for signs of depression, elder abuse, and respond to protect the vulnerable person as well as encourage the carer to obtain support. General carer issues are discussed in Chap. 1.

Photo courtesy "Love, Loss, and Laughter: Seeing Alzheimer's differently" (Greenblatt 2012)

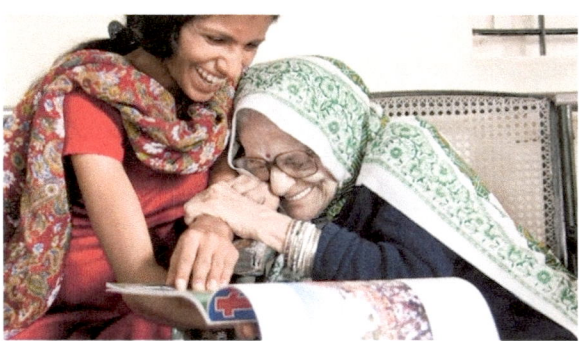

8.7.2   My Rights: At the Right Time, and in the Right Way

The current philosophical frameworks of many countries in the OECD guiding the care of older people with chronic conditions such as diabetes and dementia are underpinned by core principles that promote the individual's independence, choice where and when possible, minimise risk and focus on quality of life (Dunning et al. 2014; United Nations 2015; WHO 2016).

The National Health and Medical research (NHMRC) Partnership Centre for Dealing with Cognitive and Related Functional Decline in Older People in Australia developed Clinical Practice Guidelines and Principles of Care for People with Dementia (2016). These guidelines are underpinned by the 10 Principles of Dignity in Care, developed by the UK's Social Care Institute for Excellence. These documents complement the communication principles espoused by Alzheimer's Australia (known as Dementia Australia since October 2017) that were co-designed in consultation with people with dementia and invite people to *Talk to Me... speak clearly...avoid jargon...keep questions simple and don't question my diagnosis (as) symptoms are not always obviou*s (Alzheimer's Australia 2017a, b).

The documents emphasise the importance of respect, engaging directly with the consumer, and treating each person as an individual. The philosophy is consistent with the current trend for consumer-lead health care, greater consultation with consumers and carers, including their involvement as co-designers of organisational policy frameworks and roles such as peer-support workers, interview panels and as committee members. They are also consistent with the intent of this book.

Measuring the quality of care is important and may be more important than strictly adhering to clinical practice guidelines. Boyd et al. (2005) suggested HPs try to balance the following guidelines and adjust recommendations to suit individual's needs. The WHO Integrated Care for Older People (ICOPE) Guidelines were released in 2016 and emphasise the need...*to ensure an integrated approach focussing on 'problems' that matter most for older people, rather than specific conditions.*

The National Commission on Safety and Quality in Healthcare (2008) developed The Australian Charter of Healthcare Rights, which include the right to:

- Access (I have a right to health care)
- Safety (I have a right to safe and high quality care)
- Respect (I have a right to respect, dignity and consideration)
- Communication (I have a right to be informed about services, treatment, options and costs in a clear and open way)
- Participation (I have a right to be involved in decisions and choices about my care)
- Privacy (I have a right to privacy and confidentiality of my personal information)
- Comment (I have a right to comment on my care and to have my concerns addressed)

The charter applies to all health settings in Australia and is equally relevant globally. It enables consumers, families, carers and service providers to have a common understanding of the rights of people receiving health care. In some countries there are also legal entities such as Office of the Public Advocate in Victoria (Australia) that promote and safeguard the rights and interests of people with a disability, including investigating complaints or allegations of abuse or exploitation, providing advocacy and acting as legal guardian or appointing financial administrators to act in the vulnerable person's best interests (OPA 2017).

The Older People's Advocacy Alliance (OPAAL) UK is an organisation that promotes advocacy for older people. They offer a range of resources relevant to anyone involved in helping vulnerable adults to take decisions, make choices, manage risks and support independence. Their Support Decision tool can be used to promote choice while managing risk proportionately and realistically (2007).

These frameworks imply that people are entitled to receive information tailored to their needs and their level of understanding and that they are encouraged to participate in their care (see Chap. 2 for information about shared decision-making and older people). Therefore, it makes sense to encourage early diagnosis and develop practical and flexible treatment and care plans that individuals and their carers/representatives can adapt to suit their changing needs over the course of their illness.

For example, substitute decision-making arrangements such as Enduring Powers of Attorney for financial, legal and medical matters and Advanced Care Directives should be documented when the person has capacity to do so. Capacity assessment needs to be determined by appropriately qualified professionals, and in accordance with the legal and ethical guidelines of the country and culture the person belongs to. In the UK, a framework to decide whether someone has capacity to make specific decisions, and if not, who the designated alternative decision maker is, has been included under the Mental Health Act (The Lancet Commissions 2017).

Play to my strengths; support me; don't be afraid to be creative, and keep it real!

8.8 Real Life

It is important to note that just because a person makes a decision that could be considered 'unwise' or is contrary to a health professional's advice, does not mean that they necessarily lack capacity to give informed consent. That is, a person has a right to make bad decisions. The following vignettes describe two aged care home residents with moderate vascular dementia and diabetes whose wishes were challenged:

Val's granddaughter took her to a Dermatologist to have her dermatitis reviewed. The Dermatologist recommended a course of oral and topical steroids. The granddaughter stated that Val had always preferred naturopathic remedies and would not want to follow the specialist's recommendations. Val's GP verified the granddaughter's view because he had known Val for many years.

Some of the nursing home staff were unhappy about the suggestion to use naturopathic remedies because they believed the more orthodox medical treatment the Dermatologist recommended should be followed. A local qualified Naturopath/Aromatherapist who was also a Nurse was approached. Non-steroidal creams using essential oils were prescribed and administered after the GP clearly documented that he believed this would have been in keeping with Val's wishes in her records.

The creams took a little longer to work, the outcome was successful. The care home manager appeased the staff who objected, by providing education from the Nurse/Naturopath about the creams, and pointing out that due ethical considerations had been taken in choosing this course of action.

Both stories demonstrate a person-centred approach that considered the individual's Life Story, pre-morbid personality and weighing-up of the risks and benefits of

Dan had travelled around the roads of New Zealand for many years before vascular dementia and diet controlled type 2 diabetes made it too unsafe for him to continue to do so. He came to live closer to his eldest daughter who lived in a small country town in Australia, where he moved to the local nursing home. His hypertension grew worse, and he was advised to take anti-hypertensives to minimise stroke. He declined, as he had never liked taking medications. The GP explained to both Dan and his daughter (who had medical Enduring Power of Attorney) the risks of not taking the medication, and the nursing home manager discussed how a stroke might affect him. Dan and his daughter decided to take the risk, and he lead a comfortable life until 6 months later, a major stroke left him with a dense hemiplegia, speech and swallowing difficulties and he died 2 months later.

each situation. The individual's wishes were respected, and carers as well as primary care providers consulted.

Evidence supports the use of psychosocial and non-pharmacological interventions and a person-centred approach when faced with behavioural and psychological symptoms of dementia (BPSD). It is also considered best practice to try these techniques first. Psychotropic medications are indicated as a last resort, and at low doses for short periods of time to avoid side effects that include increased risk of falls and mortality (WHO 2012; Burns et al. 2012). Creative approaches including the role of pet and music therapy, sensory treatments such as massage, aromatherapy and learning what makes the older person happy and content is more likely to maintain equilibrium and improve their quality of life.

Connection is the energy that exists between people when they feel seen, heard and valued; when they can give and receive without judgement; and when they derive sustenance and strength from the relationship. (Brene Brown, The Gift of Imperfection 2010.)

The following are two stories that further illustrate the philosophies of a person-centred, ethically sound, realistic approach to care of the older people with diabetes and cognitive impairment.

8.9   Story 1: Wayne

8.9.1   Background

Wayne was a 65-year-old gentleman with an intellectual disability and significant hearing impairment, who had left school at age 13 and had worked for the Post Office until he was 24. He was living with his 93-year-old mother and 61-year-old brother in their own home. All three family members had been diagnosed with type 2 diabetes, Wayne most recently. His brother, John had noticed that Wayne had bilateral swollen feet, weeping leg ulcers, and was going to the toilet frequently. John encouraged Wayne to be reviewed by his GP (Wayne hadn't seen a doctor for 40 years!).

Once examined, the GP arranged for Wayne to be admitted to hospital. He was formally diagnosed with type 2 non-insulin dependent diabetes, hypertension, and he was put on a waitlist to have a large inguinal and scrotal hernia repaired. His cognition was assessed using a Mini-Mental State Examination (MMSE) with a score of 24/30, and he could read and comprehend simple instructions. In hospital, his diabetes was stabilised, treatment of his tinea and leg ulcers was commenced. He was discharged home with referrals in place for community nursing for second daily wound dressings and medication supervision, and follow-up with a GP.

8.9.2   Care Interventions

The community nurses reported that the family were living in crowded, cluttered and unhygienic conditions, and were all sleeping in lounge chairs (unable to access their bedrooms due to their apparent hoarding). They referred Wayne to a government funded community-based service where short-term case management is provided to work with the client and carers to develop a person-centred *Goal Directed Care Plan* that included a list of service contacts for Wayne, his GP and a longer-term case manager to access and share. Wayne's goals were to stay living at home, have his ulcers heal and avoid readmission to hospital. The clinicians and professional carers involved had several other concerns, but soon realised that their expectations would have to be curtailed, in keeping with Wayne's reality, circumstances and rights.

The case manager, in getting to know Wayne, identified that he was the family's food shopper and cook, and drove them all to appointments. Referrals were made for Wayne to engage with a Diabetes Nurse Educator, Dietician, Podiatrist, Audiologist, Hoarding/declutter Consultant and Pharmacist. With Wayne's agreement, and his mother's encouragement, this multi-disciplinary team provided education and support using a range of health literacy documents that were pitched at Wayne's level of understanding (Diabetes Australia Victoria 2014), calendar as an appointment diary. Capacity building and sustainability were key to promoting Wayne's self-management for the longer term.

After a few trials and errors, and a lot of practice and encouragement, Wayne mastered his blood glucometer and medication administration. The most success was had with his use of a pictorial "Healthy Eating Guide" (Novartis 2015) that used green colours and ticks indicating the best foods for his diabetes, and red colours and crosses for the foods to be discouraged. As the family shopper and cook, the changes in the family diet meant that they all benefited with more stable blood glucose levels. He successfully had his hernias repaired, enabling him to mobilise more freely, experience less discomfort and avoid complications (had he not had the operation).

Little headway was made with decluttering and cleaning but to *reduce risk*, the case manager (with the family's permission) had new smoke detectors fitted, and reported the home address to the fire brigade so that two fire units would automatically be sent to the home in the event of a fire. The beds were still unable to be accessed, so recliner chairs were purchased so the brothers could lay flatter at night, and reduce pressure load. The case manager and visiting nurses found evidence to suggest that Wayne's brother was taking financial advantage of Wayne, so steps were taken to have a Financial Administrator appointed.

Independence was encouraged, yet risks were minimised, with the philosophical guidelines of "path of least restriction" being followed (Office of the Public Advocate, Victoria).

8.10   Story 2: Elvira

8.10.1 Background

Elvira was an 86-year-old widowed lady, who had been a shopkeeper in a small country town for over 30 years until her husband died. Her family all lived in other states, so she rarely saw them and would speak with her eldest son by telephone, a few times per year. She had no active friends visiting her at the time of her transfer from a low-care hostel to a high-care dementia-specific nursing home in a bigger country town.

Elvira had been living at the hostel for 2 years because she had worsening dementia and diabetes. The staff from the hostel had limited training in dementia care, and had described Elvira as moody; she would apparently become aggressive whenever staff tried to "make her do anything she didn't want to do".

This included the staff trying to test her blood glucose levels up to four times per day. They were concerned that her moody behaviour was impacting on her blood glucose levels, and her GP had recently commenced her on insulin. Elvira was not keen on the blood glucose tests nor injections, and hostel staff had been restraining her (against the hostel's policy) to give her these. They were keen to discharge her due to her increasing verbal and physical aggression (possibly triggered by the restraint).

8.10.2 Care Interventions

The qualified and more experienced staff of the dementia-specific nursing home ascertained that Elvira had moderate dementia, with a MMSE score of 19/30 on admission. They used a *Concept Map* that documented her *abilities and needs* around Communication, Activities, Physical health, Personal Story and Personality, Environment and how her Dementia impacted on her. This was a strengths-based model, used as a foundation for her *Goal Directed Care Plan*. For example, her language skills were reasonably intact, she was prone to confabulation, had no problem-solving abilities and no short-term memory, but was easily distracted and engaged in activities she enjoyed.

The team determined that it was important for her to be allowed to settle in, and were wary of attending to too much blood glucose testing. The GP supported the team's plan to avoid stress-inducing situations, and agreed that frequent blood testing was not necessary. They would let her settle in by building trust and rapport, and learn about the things that put her in the best possible mood. There were three things that always impacted Elvira's mood positively—spending time with the dementia unit's resident cat, a rousing rendition of "Pack up Your Troubles in Your Old Kit Bag" and vanilla custard.

The staff soon learned to employ at least one of these before attempting any testing, and this usually worked. If not, they would leave her alone, but would be watching for any symptoms of hypo- or hyperglycaemia. Rather than subject Elvira to frequent blood glucose tests, the GP was comfortable with her having 3 monthly HbA1c tests (always attend to, once her good mood was established and she was likely to cooperate). He was happy for her to have a higher target for her blood glucose to avoid hypoglycaemia.

Staff soon learned that she loved to be contrary, which proved quite handy. They would say to her "I bet you can't take this tablet", or "I bet you won't let me take this little blood test"; to which she'd forcefully reply "I bet I can!". She would then (usually) either take the medication, or let the staff take the blood test.

One morning, a staff member reported to the Unit Manager that "Elvie won't put any clothes on, and is refusing to shower". The manager confirmed with the staff member that Elvira was in her own warm room, and although naked, it was deemed best to just leave her alone for the next 10 min. The staff member was advised to re-enter the room singing Elvira's favourite song, and pretending that it was the first time she'd seen her that morning.

The staff member followed this plan, and Elvira cooperated without any incident, on this second attempt. This happened on several occasions, with the same outcome. The staff concluded that she had most likely slept in the nude at home, and staff seemed more accepting of this behaviour when they considered it part of Elvira's story, and who she had always been.

About 6 months after moving to the dementia-specific home, Elvira's appetite declined and she started to lose weight, with no obvious underlying organic cause being identified. Staff had to adjust her insulin dosage accordingly, and she started to experience fluctuations in her blood glucose levels. With the advice of a Dietician and Diabetes Nurse educator, the staff provided Elvira with a mixture of food supplements, plus treats like ice-cream, cake and her favourite custard—sometimes for breakfast.

This degree of creativity and flexibility kept Elvira's mood stable, her blood glucose levels were managed, and aggressive interactions avoided. Her GP was happy because Elvira was happy, had a good quality of life, and lived happily at the home for another 6 years, passing away peacefully at the age of 96 with the resident cat snuggled next to her in bed.

8.11 Reflection Points

- Reflect on people with dementia's stories shared in the chapter. Do they reflect the key management strategies described in the introduction?
- Think about the following quote:
- *There were thousands of secrets hidden in her purse, secrets and memories that took her elsewhere. She held onto them tightly and kept them to herself. Even God did not know of them. (Suzka Collins 2016)*
- What do you think it means?
- How could you use the 'secrets hidden in her purse' to engage with the lady?
- What memories would you hide in your purse?

References

Adelman R, Tmanova L, Delgado D et al (2014) Caregiver burden: a clinical review. JAMA 311(10):1052–1059

Alzheimer's Australia (2017a) Key facts and statistics www.fightdementia.org.au/statistics. Accessed Sept 2017

Alzheimer's Australia (2017b) Support for carers. A practical guide to services for families and friends of people with dementia. www.fightdementia.org.au/support-for-carers.pdf. Accessed Sept 2017

Alzheimer's Australia Tasmania (2017) "This is Me—Life Story Book". www.fightdementia.org. au. Accessed Jul 2017

Alzheimer's Disease International (2013) The global impact of dementia 2013–2050: policy brief for heads of Government. Alzheimer's Disease International, London

Alzheimer's Disease International (2015) World Alzheimer report 2015: The Global impact of dementia—an analysis of prevalence, Incidence, Costs and Trends.

Australian Commission on Safety and Quality in Healthcare (2008) www.safetyandquality.gov.au/national-priorities/charterof-healthcare-rights Australian Government

Biessels GJ, Strachan MW, Visseren FL, Kappelle LJ, Whitmer RA (2014) Dementia and cognitive decline in type 2 diabetes and prediabetic stages: towards targeted interventions. Lancet Diabet Endocrinol 2:246–255

de Boer I, Sun W, Gao X et al (2014) DCCT/EDIC Research Group. Effect of intensive diabetes treatment on albuminuria in type 1 diabetes: long-term follow-up of the Diabetes Control and

Complications Trial and Epidemiology of Diabetes Interventions and Complications study. Lancet Diabet Endocrinol 2:793–800

Bourgeois M, Dijkstra K, Hickey E (2005) Impact of communicative interaction on meaningful quality of life in dementia. J Med Speech Lang Pathol 13:37–50

Boyd C, Darer J, Boult C (2005) Clinical practice guidelines and quality of care for older patients with multiple comorbid diseases. JAMA 294(6):716–724

Burns K, Jayasinha R, Tsang R, Brodaty H (2012) Behaviour management—a guide to good practice: managing behavioural and psychological symptoms of dementia (BPSD). Australian Government's Department of Health and Ageing. http://www.dementiaresearch.org.au/images/dcrc/output-files/328-.2012_dbmas_bpsd_guidelines_guide.pdf

Ciudin A, Simo-Serva O, Hernandez C et al (2017) Retinal microperimtry: a new tool for identifying type 2 diabetic patients at risk of developing Alzheimer's disease. Diabetes 66(12):3098–3104. https://doi.org/10.2337/db173-0

Collins English Dictionary (2011) Harper Collins

Collins S (undated) Meet Suzka Collins, author of "Wonders in Dementialand"—AlzAuthors. https://alzauthors.com/2017/.../meet-suzka-collins-author-of-wonders-in-dementialand

Diabetes Australia Victoria (2014) Pictorial guides—healthy eating, my feet and diabetes, managing my diabetes, exercise and diabetes

Dunning T, Duggan N, Savage S (2014) The McKellar guidelines for managing older people in residential and other care settings. Centre for Nursing and Allied Health Research Deakin University and Barwon Health, Geelong

Fisher C (2017) Mental health disorders and dementia Presentation given at

Geerlings M, Bouter L, Schoevers R et al (2000) Depression and risk of cognitive decline and Alzheimer's disease. The British Journal of Psychiatry 176(6):568–575

Gill, Dr Thomas in Grubin, David (2015) "Rx: The Quiet Revolution" documentary. Accessed Jul 2017

Girdwain J (2011) Gray area—who will treat aging boomers? Aging Well 4(4):30

Greenblatt C (2012) Love, loss, and laughter: seeing Alzheimer's differently. Lyons Press, Guilford, CT

Hafner K (2016) As population ages, where are the Geriatricians? In New York Times. Accessed 25 Jan 2016

Hertzog C, Kramer AF, Wilson RS, Lindenberger U (2009) Enrichment effects on adult cognitive development: can the functional capacity of older adults be preserved and enhanced? Psychol Sci Publ Interest. 9:1–65

Hill J (2015) Diabetes and dementia: the implications or diabetes nursing. J Diabet Nurs 19(4):2015

International Psychogeriatric Association (1996) report on the international consensus conference on behavioural disturbances of dementia, Washington DC, March 31–April 2, 1996.

International Psychogeriatric Association (2002) BPSD: Introduction to behavioural and psychological symptoms of dementia. http://www.ipa-online.org

Jampolsky GJ (2000) Teach only love: the twelve principles of attitudinal healing. Beyond Words Publishing, Hillsboro, OR

Lipska K et al (2013) HbA1c and risk of severe hypoglycemia in type 2 diabetes. Diabet Care 36(11):3535–3542. https://doi.org/10.2337/dc13-0610

Marseglia A, Fratiglioni L, Laukka EJ, Santoni G, Pedersen NL, Backman L, Weili X (2016) Early cognitive deficits in Type 2 diabetes: a population-based study. J Alzheimers Dis 53(3):1069–1078

McCrimmon RJ, Ryan CM, Frier BM (2012) Diabetes and cognitive dysfunction. Lancet 379:2291–2299

National Health & Medical Research Council (NHMRC) Partnership Centre for Dealing with Cognitive and Related Functional Decline in Older People (2016) Clinical practice guidelines and principles of care for people with dementia

NICE (2010) Dementia quality standard QS1. NICE, London. www.nice.org.uk/qs1. Accessed Jun 2017

Novartis (2015) A guide to healthy food choice, pictorial wheel. http://swapit.gov.au/ways-to-swap/food-swap-suggester

Office of the Public Advocate, Victoria, Australia (2017) www.publicadvocate.vic.gov.au/disability. Accessed Aug 2017

Older People's Advocacy Alliance (OPAAL) UK (2007) Support Decision Tool Independence, "Choice and Risk: a guide to best practice in supported decision making" 21 May 2007, UK Department of Health

Puttanna A, Padinjakara NK (2017) Management of diabetes and dementia. Br J Diabet 17(3).

Rapport L (2017) Older adults more likely to disclose suicidal thoughts as they age. http://bit.ly/2xPHPZ

Rock P, Roiser J, Riedel W et al (2013) Cognitive impairment and depression: a systematic review and meta-analysis. Psychol Med 29:1–12

Sinclair AJ, Gadsby R, Hillson R, Forbes A, Bayer AJ (2013) Brief report: use of mini-cog as a screening tool for cognitive impairment in diabetes primary care. Diabet Res Clin Pract 100(1):23–25

Sinclair AJ, Hillson R, Bayer AJ (2014) Diabetes and dementia in older people: best practice statement by a multidisciplinary National Expert Working Group. Diabet Med 31(9):1024–1031

Sinclair AJ, Dunning T, Rodriguez-Manas L (2015) Diabetes in older people: new insights and remaining challenges. Lancet Diabet Endocrinol 3(4):275–285

The Lancet Commission on Dementia Prevention, Intervention, and Care (2017) www.thelancet.com. Published online July 20, 2017. doi: https://doi.org/10.1016/S0140-6736(17)31363-6

The Royal Australasian College of Physicians (RACP) and Australian & New Zealand Society for Geriatric Medicine (ANZSGM) (2012) Response to the questions on notice, house standing committee on health and ageing inquiry into dementia: early diagnosis and intervention August 2012. p. 1–4

Training, Research and Education for Nurses in Diabetes (TREND UK) with Institute of Diabetes for Older People (IDOP) (2013) Diabetes and dementia—guidance on practical management. instituteofdiabetes.org. Accessed 16 Oct 2013

United Nations (2015) World population ageing 1950—2050 report, population division, department of economic and social affairs

Velayudhan L, Poppe M, Archer N, Proitsi P, Brown R, Lovestone S (2009) Risk of developing dementia in people with diabetes and mild cognitive impairment. Br J Psychiatry 196(1):36–40

World Health Organization (WHO) (2015) World report on ageing and health. WHO, Geneva

World Health Organization (WHO) (2016) Integrated Care for Older People (ICOPE) guidelines in www.thelancetonline.com, vol 387. Accessed 9 Jan 2016

World Health Organization (WHO) and Alzheimer's Disease International (2012) Dementia: a public health priority. World Health Organization, Geneva

The Art of Using Technology to Personalise Care with Older People with Diabetes

9

Natalie Wischer and Leanne Mullan

> *Before you become too entranced with gorgeous gadgets and mesmerizing video displays, let me remind you that information is not knowledge, knowledge is not wisdom, and wisdom is not foresight. Each grows out of the other, and we need them all.*
>
> *(Arthur C. Clarke)*

Key Points

- Diabetes is well suited to digital interventions.
- Older people are capable of using technology.
- Technologies should be simple to use and fit into the lifestyle and resources of the person.
- Technologies should offer solutions and remove barriers to existing problems.
- Technologies should be integrated with and complement the existing lifestyle and drug treatments of individuals with diabetes
- Validation matters! Work with and support the older person with diabetes to use technology.

N. Wischer (✉)
Australian Diabetes Online Services, Sydney, NSW, Australia

Monash University, Clayton, VIC, Australia
e-mail: ceo@nadc.net.au

L. Mullan
National Association of Diabetes Centres and Australian Diabetes Society (ADS), Sydney, NSW, Australia
e-mail: leanne.mullan@nadc.net.au

© Springer International Publishing AG, part of Springer Nature 2018
T. Dunning (ed.), *The Art and Science of Personalising Care with Older People with Diabetes*, https://doi.org/10.1007/978-3-319-74360-8_9

9.1   Introduction and Overview

Marj's smiling eyes and timeworn face were *almost* enough to suppress my internal sigh. Not many people brought their blood glucose meters to their appointments today. Marj was the third person who did not bring her meter to her appointment. But, before I had a chance to explain the value of being able to see how her blood glucose levels responded to a multitude of factors, Marj plunged her old hands into her oversized handbag, fumbled around for a while, and pulled out her smart phone.

I presumed she wanted to showcase the latest photos of her grandchildren: instead, almost bursting with pride, Marj showed me how she had been recording her blood glucose levels, insulin doses, food intake and exercise on a diabetes app on to her phone. I couldn't hide my surprise. The oldest person on my appointment list for the day introduced me to a glucose tracking application (app)! From that moment on I was hooked. My preconceived perception of technology use was transformed. I realised that older people do indeed use technology! An old dog (me) was definitely taught a new trick!

Digital technologies are rapidly changing the healthcare landscape. Society struggles to keep pace with technological advances that move faster than the National Broadband Network (NBN) in Australia. Yet enthusiasm is building for the potential health solutions technology it will bring. Technology enables faster and simpler ways to collect and share information/data as well as streamlining ways to connect people. Technology is changing the way we communicate to promote better outcomes for people living with diabetes.

Health professionals (HP) and the general public seek health information using assorted technologies. There is a growing trend towards using technology to help HPs help individuals manage their health. Conversely, there is the expectation for individuals to be able to almost instantly connect with their healthcare team. Whilst the person with diabetes can benefit from advancing technologies, HPs face challenges as they endeavour to keep up with new information and digital therapies. Whilst HPs attempt to limit the digital knowledge divide, they are also left responsible for ensuring the 'latest' and 'greatest' gadgets add value and do not detract from care goals.

Becker Healthcare (2013) surveyed 7000 participants and found 60% said they would monitor their chronic disease using a mobile phone application and 90% said they would use a technology service that enabled them to ask a clinician a question. The survey thus suggested that approximately 500 million people globally would use a healthcare app in the following year. These data are remarkable, particularly when many older people can remember, all too clearly, a time before the mobile phone.

There is great optimism about the positive influence of connectivity and the development and integration of new care delivery models that can promote personalised care and improve outcomes at a lower cost, particularly for older Australians who often experience social isolation due to physical limitations and distance. The Nielsen Panorama survey (2007–2008) showed 46% of older internet users accessed information about medical-related topics and services, which indicates that the impact of healthcare technology was evident over 10 years ago.

This chapter investigates technology use amongst older people and reflects on global statistics and research. It explores the benefits of technology use for older people and unravels some of the challenges to technology uptake. Various technology options are discussed to provide an overview of the expansive technology options accessible today and those expected to become mainstream in the future, including devices to help people move, be safe at home and improve the health of older people whilst remaining in their own home. Further, the key elements of 'successful' technology use is identified using practical examples and suggestions for how HPs can apply the suggestions in their practice. In addition, advice about how to overcome technology challenges will be described to help readers understand the use of newer technologies for older people living with diabetes.

For the purpose of the chapter 'technology' is defined as tool that has been developed to solve a problem.

9.2   Demographic Data

On a recent visit to a technology retail outlet I observed eight older people sitting with their devices receiving a lesson on the basics of tablet use. These older people appeared to be highly engaged, asking questions, chatting to one another and laughing. I was taken aback by my subconscious surprise at seeing older people engaged with a device and socialising.

In the past, computer, smart phone and internet was associated with younger age, statistically and in societal attitudes. However, from the real example cited on page xx negative ageist attitudes and stereotypes remain today, despite a growing number of reports that indicate technology use amongst older people is on the rise.

The World Health Organisation (WHO) (2015) identified that the proportion of the world's populations aged over 60 will increase from 12% in 2015 to 22% in 2050, which indicates there will be over 2 billion people older than the age of 60 within the next 35 years.

In early 2017 there were 3.8 billion internet users, 4.9 billion unique mobile phone users and 2.8 billion active social media users globally (Kemp 2017). In just one year, there was a 21% increase in social media users and mobile phones have overtaken laptops and desktops, and now using 50% of the web traffic (Kemp 2017). The Pew Research Centre (2012) reported that internet use among people aged older than 64 increased by 150% between 2009 and 2011. The Australian Bureau of Statistics (ABS) (2016) reported that 51% (3,873,000 Australians) older than 65 years used the internet in the previous 12 months. That's a lot of connected older people!

Despite these data, internet and technology use declines with age (Pew Research Centre 2017). Smartphone ownership doubled in America between 2013 and 2017, however, uptake amongst those people 65 and older still lags behind the overall population: almost half of all older people own a smartphone, a third own a tablet, a third use social media and two-thirds access the internet (Pew Research Centre 2017). Likewise, nearly 45% of Australians older than 85 years do not have home internet access compared to a mere 7% people aged 55 years or younger. Internet connectivity and age remain inversely related.

9.3   What Impacts on Technology Uptake in Older People?

Several factors influence technology use beside age. These include some demographic factors. For example, men exhibit higher levels of internet use than women (Chesters et al. 2013). Further, people with higher education levels utilise technology more than those with lower levels of education. Research indicates that 87% of older people with a university degree access the internet compared to 40% who did not attend university (Chesters et al. 2013).

In addition, a US study found the annual household income also influenced internet connectivity: 90% of older people with an annual household income greater than $75,000 utilise the internet and 82% have access to the internet at home (Pew Research Centre 2014). The proportion with home internet access declines significantly amongst older people earning less than $30,000 annually, with only 39% accessing the internet and 25% having an internet connection at home (Pew Research Centre 2014).

Furthermore, physical abilities and limitations could also impact on technology uptake in older people. Dexterity, sight, motor function, coordination and cognition can change during the lifespan and impact on a person's ability to use certain forms of technology effectively.

9.4   Technology Benefits

Some of the undisclosed benefits of technology use are: connection to others, which alleviates social isolation, gaining knowledge, and simplifying and personalising life (Feist and McDougall 2013). It is easy to assume technologies are not applicable to older people due to a lack of exposure; however a recent study amongst patients aged 65 and older with a history of a cardiac event found 74% were willing to participate in a technology-based healthcare and support program (Neubeck et al. 2015). Neubeck et al. (2015) also identified that at least 67% accessed the internet and more than 50% used a mobile phone to assist with their healthcare. Likewise Chow et al. (2015) showed well-designed, simple technologies can improve patient outcomes. For example, a systematic review of 17 randomised control trials ($N = 25,101$) found that automated messaging interventions almost doubled the odds that people would adhere to their cardio-metabolic medications compared to usual care (Kassavou and Sutton 2017). Further, a recent mobile phone texting program ($n = 710$), whereby patients in the intervention group ($n = 352$) received four text messages per week for 6 months in addition to usual care found the use of lifestyle focussed text messaging resulted in improved LDL cholesterol and improvements in other cardiovascular disease risk factors (Chow et al. 2015). The text messages in this program provided advice, motivational reminders and support to change lifestyle behaviours.

Newer technologies provide a forum for communication regardless of the person's location and can help offset loneliness and isolation. Feist and McDougall (2013) undertook a study in Victoria, Australia ($n = 48$), and found the self-rated well-being score of those connected through technology was higher than those who were not connected (64% versus 58% respectively). Technology can empower people by enabling them access to information regardless of their mobility level.

Feist and McDougall (2013) undertook a self-rated survey that was completed pre and post a technology integration pilot study, known as the 'Linking Rural Older People to Community through Technology' Project (LROP). The study enabled the use of new technologies by older people and observed and recorded personal interaction with the new technology. Eighty nine percentage of the 48 participants stated their access to information improved and 72% said they felt more independent, better informed and their ability to stay in touch with family and friends improved compared with those who did not use technology.

Evidence also shows that technology enhances health outcomes related to technology use. A recent meta-analysis, mostly concerning apps for type 2 diabetes, demonstrated a reduction in glycosylated haemoglobin (HbA1c) of 0.49% compared with control groups (Victorian Health Promotion Foundation 2013). Feist and McDougall (2013) also identified health benefits and demonstrated a marked increase in the proportion of participants rating their health as excellent or very good from 16% pre-pilot to more than 40% post-pilot. This highlights the positive effect of engagement through the use of technologies on health and well-being of older people. These results were recorded by the 'Linking Rural Older People to Community through Technology' (LROP) project as outlined above.

Several reports provide insight into the many technological solutions available to the older person at home. These include safety and security measures including falls detection technology, mobility aids, smoke monitors and door locks. Personal emergency response systems contribute to independent living and safety (Stokke 2016). Readily available technology-driven treatment support being used includes health monitoring systems and programs, medication compliance alerts and telemedicine services. Social connectedness through mobile phones, video, email and text messaging are further examples of technological benefits for older people (Bouma et al. 2009).

In Japan, where more than 25% of the population is older than 64 years of age (McCurry 2015), there has been a move to produce robots to assist people with dementia by alleviating social isolation and improving safety in the home. Robotic devices are being developed that can assist with activities of daily living such as bathing. Robots can assist with toileting, bathing, social interaction, personal mobility, monitoring and therapeutics (The Conversation 2017).

Further research is underway to develop smart clothing that can collect a diverse range of indicators such as heart rate, movement, oximetry, temperature, and exercise data including stride length, cadence and ground contact time. Smart clothing entering the market has Bluetooth connectivity and links to companion applications. Some clothing has inbuilt vibrations that gently pulse parts of the body to encourage movement. Socks are available that can detect pressure and foot complications before they actually occur. Fitted with Global Positioning Systems (GPS), ultra violet and breathing sensors and wearable health monitoring devices such as watches will have a huge impact on future healthcare, and when affordable, will influence the way the care for older people is tailored and personalised.

In addition, ambient assisted living technology where sensors, physiological signals and home environment monitoring can notify HPs, relatives and carers about changes or abnormalities are emerging (Chen et al. 2016). The video-based sensing and pattern analysis accompanied by internet technology could assist HP to monitor

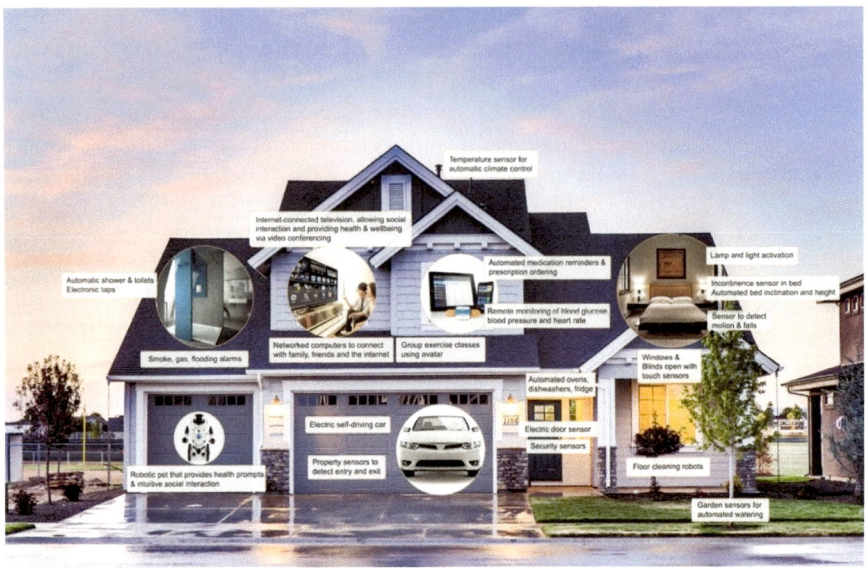

Fig. 9.1 Image adapted from Smart Technologies for Older People—a systematic literature review of smart technologies that promote health and well-being of older people living at home. The University of Melbourne & Institute for a Broadband Enabled Society, 2012

and assess the older person in their home. Such technology obviously requires financial investment, which could be a limitation for many older people with diabetes. Also on the other end of the monitoring system, trained health professionals are needed to effectively and safely interpret and respond to the diversity of the incoming data. This also requires financial investment both in equipment and human resources. Privacy may also be a concern for the older person as information is transmitted via the internet where security issues exist and can be questioned, see Fig. 9.1.

9.5   Challenges to Uptake by Older Adults

As discussed, a number of factors facilitate or prevent older people from using technology, in addition to mention the HPs' own attitudes and beliefs. The ageing process is accompanied with physical changes that include decline in dexterity, mobility, cognition, some aspects of memory, hearing and eyesight (see Chap. 1). Psychological factors also have an impact on technology usage and attitudes influence whether the individual will adopt new technology. Many older people feel the internet does not have any relevance to their lives. Some beliefs are:

New technologies are changing too fast for me to keep up
and
I'm too old to learn about new technology

This suggests technology may not be suitable for everybody. An Australian Communications and Media Authority (ACMA) Consumer Survey ($n = 1637$),

(2008) found more than 50% of respondents over the age of 65 years self-rated their internet competency as below average, which could affect technology uptake.

Financial costs can also make it difficult for older people to afford technology. Internet connection rates are lower for people who live alone, outside capital city areas or who have a low income. Over 80% of people 65 years and older live independently: an estimated 40% to 50% live in lone-person households (Australian Academy of Technological Sciences and Engineering (ATSE) 2010). Older people are more likely to have a lower household income than younger people (Feist and McDougall 2013), which illustrates the inequities that exist between younger and older people.

The age-related technological inequity can be apparent between parents and their children and is even more apparent in older people who have left employment before technology use became prevalent. Further, older people tend not to live with their children and do not have the same exposure to new technologies.

Aaron Smith from the Pew Research Centre (2014) found a lack of adequate assistance was a challenge to technology uptake. The Pew Research Center's Internet Project July 18–September 30, 2013 tracking survey identified that only 18% of older people in the study ($n = 1801$) felt comfortable learning to use a new device such as a smartphone or tablet on their own, while 77% indicated they would need someone to help 'walk them through the process'. In addition, cost, denial of need, lack of interest and fear were barriers to accessing the internet for some older people.

9.6   Technology Options

9.6.1   Cloud Connected Glucose Monitoring Systems

A range of blood glucose meters as well as other devices such as blood pressure monitors, pulse oximeters, scales and ECG devices that enable results to be stored and accessed in the 'cloud' are available. Essentially, cloud storage means that, once the data are recorded, anyone with approved access can review the results remotely. Bluetooth and cloud technology enable people to share information with family, friends and/or HPs, which can facilitate timely feedback on the required health interventions.

Some tablet-based health applications are used to support older people to be cared for at home. Such tablets can be linked with a range of Bluetooth-enabled devices to upload biometric data with a healthcare organisation such as the Royal District Nursing Service or private health providers. Staff within the healthcare organisation can review the uploaded data and provide prompt feedback. Many of these devices also have the option for telehealth connections to be hosted between the person in their home and their HPs. Medication reminders, automated ordering of pharmaceuticals and other useful health apps are also available on a number of these remote home monitoring systems.

Each morning Beryl follows the same routine: she weighs herself, checks her blood pressure, pulse, oxygen saturation, then blood glucose levels. All of this information is uploaded onto her home monitoring tablet and securely transmitted to a central location and checked by a nurse. Beryl has diabetes, chronic obstructive pulmonary disease, hypertension, and early signs of dementia. She wants to live independently in her home for as long as possible.

Beryl may receive a phone call if any clinical parameters are out of her target range set by her and her GP. When she has had low blood glucose for example, the nurse calls her via the video conferencing app available in the workplace to discuss her treatment of the hypoglycaemic episode, as well as check that she is okay. The telehealth consultation also enables HPs to provide opportunistic guidance, education and reinforce self-management practices in a timely manner.

Beryl checks the list of her morning medication after she performs her morning routines. She swallows her tablets, self-administers her insulin and then taps the screen again to acknowledge that she followed her morning medication regimen. She noticed that her metformin supply was running low. She then touched the appropriate box on the screen to select metformin from the list, and her script is automatically filled. It will be ready for her to collect from her selected pharmacy later that day. An estimated 50% of medicines are not taken as prescribed; therefore, it is evident that the pharmaceutical reminder system could have a significant impact on medication adherence and therefore disease outcomes.

Beryl receives an alert reminding her of her upcoming podiatrist appointment just before she begins to Google for a gift for her granddaughter on her home monitoring tablet. She checks her calendar. She is grateful for the reminder because she has a tendency to forget some of her appointments. The system helps her remember to attend these.

9.6.2   Telehealth Services

Although telehealth is no longer a new technology, it continues to be popular and provides useful healthcare option, especially for older people. The convenience of connecting with specialist healthcare providers from one's home or local general practice can make an enormous difference by reducing the burden of cost, time and the stress of travelling to health appointments in less familiar areas. Most general practices, particularly those located in rural and remote regions, now offer telehealth connectivity to specialists. Further, there is a growing range of telehealth services that can be used from one's own home, including access to online general practitioners and other specialist health providers. Finding local service providers with telehealth options can be as simple as a Google search.

9.6.3   Education Services

Often when we think of education, we may picture a traditional class room or group-based setting with someone teaching the content. Technology is changing the way education and information is provided.

The number and type of online support and type 2 diabetes prevention programs available is increasing rapidly. There is a range of programs based on the landmark National Diabetes Prevention Program (DPP) (2002); others are designed to be tailored to the needs of the individual who enrols and their particular age, demographic and health requirements as well as their health literacy.

9.6.4   Service Support Tools

I once met an orthopaedic surgeon who used a range of technologies to provide pre- and post-operative support to his patients. He designed a range of picture-based print outs as well as video clips with audio instructions that he could tailor into an exercise package for each individual based on their needs and learning styles. Even making and getting to an appointment was improved by technology. His online booking system showed the person the quickest way to get to the clinic depending on the time and day of the booking and also had a link for someone to arrange a taxi or an Uber to pick them up to make it to the appointment on time (conversation with Warkentine on June 10, 2014)

HPs may feel they can only dream of having access to such tools, but most are now readily available. Website development is as easy as creating a Word document and pricing is now very low. Developing resources or links to reputable websites is a highly effective tool for increasing the quality and usability of educational support.

9.6.5   Mobile Apps

There is no shortage of choice of mobile apps for diabetes and other health conditions. However, finding evidenced-based and high quality apps is the key. Unfortunately, there are very few clinically validated apps available but it is expected this may change in the future. Approved apps such as the Food and Drug Administration (FDA) approved Blue Star app in the United States improves HbA1c by up to 1.3% (Quinn et al. 2011). This app and others are beginning to show promise as being impactful in diabetes management. For this reason, it is important for health professionals to be aware of this popular avenue for health advice and support. For HPs the rules for finding useful and reputable mobile apps for older people are no different from the rules for all technology. Review and research what users say about the app, find out who developed it, for example, was it developed by a commercial firm or a HP? Does it synchronise with other devices the person is using. Is it easy to use, and most importantly does it offer a solution to a problem or an issue the person has?

One app designed specifically for older people is the Five.Good.Friends app, which aims to match those living at home to nearby service providers that may be able to assist them in their daily activities. The Australian app developer, Simon Lockyer, designed the app in the hope that it may assist people to remain in their homes for longer. He wanted to find a way to enhance the connections and support being provided to older people in their homes as he had an understanding of the value of relationships in the health of older people. The app connects older people with skilled workers, carers, family members and companions. Such apps are becoming more readily accessible and available to older people living at home, providing HPs with another avenue to explore with the older person with diabetes, to optimise support and connection.

9.6.6 Text Messaging

Short Messaging Service, otherwise known as SMS, has been available on most phones since the mid-1980s; therefore SMS is a familiar tool to mobile users. SMS has been used in healthcare education and support across the world (Ramachandran et al. 2013). Many third world countries use SMS to provide support and information because it is low cost and mobile phones have a high rate of ownership, even in low income populations.

A number of benefits of SMS messaging demonstrate lifestyle improvements, whilst SMS is also seen as an acceptable form of communication (Holmes 2011). It can also be used for appointment and medication reminders and HPs can set up automated systems that deliver these messages, which are inexpensive and readily available.

9.6.7 Wearable Activity Trackers

There is increasing research on the benefits of wearable fitness trackers. Most indicate they are only successful for people who are already motivated and will not remain a long-term partner in most peoples' health toolkit (Jakicic et al. 2016). However, it is important to note that these devices can provide useful insights into a person's normal activity and sleep profiles, even when they are only worn for a short time. Piwek et al. (2016) suggest summarises that wearables can provide personalised health data that could assist with behavioural change interventions.

There is a vast array of activity trackers on the market that range from basic to highly sophisticated. When purchasing a device HPs can recommend older people with diabetes/families choose a simple to use tracker with clear, large, easy-to-read screens. A device that just shows step counts may provide some encouragement and motivation and these are cheap and available in a large variety of stores. More sophisticated devices that monitor sleep and synchronise with other tracking and monitoring devices can also be considered but a commitment and interest should be demonstrated before investing additional income into these, and therefore starting at the simple and low cost end of the wearable device market is highly recommended.

9.7 Machine Learning

Machine learning is not new or futuristic. It is an extension of artificial intelligence (AI) and the first known machine learnt program was developed by Arthur Samuel in 1956 who developed a computer system that learnt how to beat him in checkers. In normal computing, machines are coded so as to perform a certain way following algorithms, but in machine learning the computer is designed to teach itself. The more data received, the 'smarter' it becomes. Scary? Yes! Useful? Absolutely! Examples can be seen in the way Facebook structures posts and advertising to individual people, how dating apps find the closest match and how Amazon may find you the book you would most likely wish to read without you even entering anything into the search function.

Machine learning is no stranger in healthcare and is being used across the spectrum of diabetes care. Diabetes prevention and management programs are using chatbots which are where artificial intelligence driven conversational programs simulate a human voice and conversation. An example of this can be seen in the My Diabetes Coach system developed by a team at the University of Melbourne.

Artificial intelligence is also used in meter and pump technologies and predictive analysis of complications. This technology is exciting in that it can learn more about a person over time and tailor outputs specifically for the individual. Add to this the benefits of 'Big Data', an extremely large data set that is designed to analyse trends over time, we can expect significant advancements in not only diabetes care but the healthcare sector as a whole.

9.8   Key Elements of Success

Given that technology use amongst older people is still lower than among younger people, how can HPs promote technology-related health success stories to the older people they care for and support? There are several key elements for success: personalisation, simplicity, education/support and connection.

9.8.1   Personalising

One of the key elements of ensuring technology use assists the older person is to ensure the type of technology used and adopted is personalised for the individual. Personal relevance of technology is a major driver and will directly correlate with use (Feist and McDougall 2013). Many people have downloaded an application they thought looked great. It was free, had great reviews and it promised to make life easier. Once they started to probe the features of the app and information within it, they realised it was not going to help them. Within 5 min, the app was uninstalled and life went on without it.

As with all interventions, it is critical to understand a person's motivation, situation and needs. What do they want to achieve? One person may simply want to be able to connect with their diabetes educator or specialist quickly, share blood glucose readings. Another may want to participate in a home exercise program or connect to others in their homes via the internet to enhance socialisation.

Another person may want assistance to calculate carbohydrate intake or to discover the impact of 'doing the gardening' on their diabetes. Older adults often adopt new technologies so they can: '…Catch up with kids and grandchildren', '…Keep my brain active' or '…Know what is going on in the world'. The value of personal relevance is always fundamental to whether people adopt new technologies—indeed whether they adopt new 'anything'.

Discovering the person's motivation, values, preferences and health goals and personalising technology to support activities that are meaningful for that person improves outcomes and paves the way to success. If an individual recognises a specific need, they are more motivated to find a solution, answer or tool to assist with their problem—the solution may very well come in the form of technology! (Chap. 2 discusses personalising care and shared decision-making and Chap. 3 outline the knowledge skills and competence HPS need to be effective.)

9.8.2 Top Tips for Personalising Care Using Technology

Before suggesting any technology, important points to consider include the following and they should be discussed with the older person and or their families and other carers:

- Which technology would help the older person to meet their goals?
- What tools would be most helpful for the older person?
- Why are you suggesting technology—what are the aims?
    - Is it to alleviate social isolation? (e.g. virtual exercise group, social network group)
    - Is it for health monitoring? (e.g. assessing and monitoring blood glucose levels, or the effect of the introduction of a new medication)
    - Is it to improve safety through a personal alarm or environmental monitoring? (i.e. older person with hypoglycaemic unawareness).
- The equipment the older person has—do they have a smart phone / tablet or personal computer?
- Internet connectivity—does the older person have internet access at home?
- What is the financial impact of the technology?
- Is the older person familiar with the type of technology?
- Is the older person confident with the technology?
- Can the older person troubleshoot if required?
- What supports do they have available in uptaking new technology?
- Are there any barriers to the use of technology:
    - Fear of personal information sharing (data security)?
    - Does the older person have any physical limitations that need consideration in adopting new technology (e.g. dexterity, vision or hearing impairment)?
    - Language difficulties/health literacy/literacy?
    - Will there be financial limitations in the use of technology?
    - Are there issues of cognitive capacity?

When personalising technology options for the older person, financial considerations must be made. This includes not only the initial start-up cost, for example, purchasing a smart phone or tablet, but also ongoing costs, such as internet connections, software, updates and repair. The individual's physical abilities and limitations should also be factored when choosing which technology may be able to assist them in achieving their goals. Dexterity, sight, motor function, coordination and cognition should be taken into account. It is good to remember that most smartphones, tablets and computers have settings that allow for increased font size, applications for reading text aloud, and improved background lighting for increased readability.

9.8.3   Simplicity

Many people have encountered situations where they have been given a lot of new information quickly, presented in an unfamiliar or suboptimal way, which has resulted in very little of the information being retained. Memories of my first guitar lesson spring to mind, as I left the lesson with sore fingers and feeling as though I would never get the hang of it. So it is with introducing health technology. Effective communication, encouragement and simple messages are the core of person-centred care.

There is increasing evidence that indicates simple and well-designed technology can improve diabetes outcomes. A recent systematic review of 14 randomised controlled trials concluded that apps can be as effective as an adjuvant intervention in routine diabetes self-management interventions (Victorian Health Promotion Foundation 2013). The researchers also concluded that most application interventions reviewed were simple to use, had nominal cost and were likely to be effective at a population level.

After establishing the motivations and goals of the individual and considering how to personalise the technology, start with simple activities that are meaningful to the individual such as using email or entering blood glucose levels into an internet-based program. Utilise clean and simple devices and programs and provide similar straightforward explanations. Choose devices or programs that are easy to set up, plug and play and ensure that all programs are credible and work well. An evaluation of patient engagement, quality and safety of 1046 healthcare-related patient-focussed applications for chronic disease found only 43% (iOS) and 27% (android) were actually likely to be useful (Singh et al. 2016). This finding highlights to needs to ensure the particular device or program chosen is reliable, useful and meets the individual's needs.

Some individuals may like to experiment with the technology whereas others would like succinct accurate instructions. Research supports the notion that many people learn best by doing rather than watching or listening (REF), so work with the individual, allow them to practice, be hands on, troubleshoot and ask questions, and, importantly, listen to the answers.

9.9   Education and Support

On average it takes more than 2 months before a new behaviour becomes automatic (habit). Habit forming varies widely depending on the type of behaviour (e.g. motor/rote), the individual and the surrounding circumstances and their cognition. It can take anywhere from 18 to 254 days to develop a habit (Lally et al. 2010). Therefore, it is important for health professionals to provide consistent regular education and contact when introducing a person to a new health technology. Having regular catch up review sessions with an individual, especially during the learning phase, will assist them to feel confident to use the technology so it becomes habitual and part of business as usual.

Various forms of education can be provided. Some individuals may thrive on a self-directed and work at their own pace, others may enjoy learning in a small group of similar aged older people. Others may blossom in larger group learning situations and succeed in part due to the socialisation and support from other individuals (peer learning/shared learning and problem-solving). Whether education and learning is completed one-on-one, in groups or with in-home support, it is vital to the successful uptake of technology to provide opportunities for ongoing learning, support, reiteration and contact with HPs and support networks, such as fellow learners, family and friends.

Magnusson et al. (2004) stated that older people's negative attitudes toward technology services can possibly be altered if they receive appropriate and focussed training that meets their individual learning needs and provides potential benefits to support them. Suitable and tailored technology education can increase self-esteem and improve well-being (Leavengood 2001; Furlong 1995). Ensuring education and support is provided in a non-threatening environment will also be vital to success as well as the utilisation of specifically designed technology education and support resources.

Electronic brain training puzzles or games may also assist the older person to learn and retain new skills, as they are said to increase blood flow to the prefrontal cortex (the areas important to thought and memory). Studies indicate that supervised brain training may lead to small improvements in memory, reasoning, problem-solving and thinking in similar tasks in older people (Simons et al. 2016; Nouchi et al. 2012). Several other studies, however, do not show benefits of brain training puzzles in learning and retaining new skills. HPs need to consider the individual and their learning style and capacity when developing education and support plans.

9.10   Connection

Many health technology programs provide real-time tracking, social features and cloud-based communication, thus connection is easier than in the past. Maintaining connection with individuals can provide an extra layer of motivation, support and encouragement as people embark on a new journey of technological discovery. As discussed earlier in the chapter, social isolation is common amongst older people and promoting socialisation with others through internet-based streams can improve psychological well-being.

It is important to regularly evaluate how the technology is helping or hindering the individual as part of personalised care and continuous improvement and to enable appropriate modifications to be made when necessary to suit each individual. Success relies on identifying and addressing any challenges the individual encounters using the technology as soon as possible. Working with the individual to discuss outcomes achieved using the new technology such as behaviour change and improved diabetes management can be part of the evaluation process. Remember the outcomes and goals achieved may vary between the HP and the individual. For example, the older person with diabetes may not have had any improvements in clinical outcomes, such as an improvement in HbA1c, but they may feel less socially isolated due to the connection gained through the use of a new device or technology. Some individuals may thrive on an inbuilt reward system and working together to find strategies that personalise the experience for each individual could promote success.

With all the distraction of the bright and shiny newer devices, we should pause for a moment to remember that even the humble stethoscope is a piece of technology and was touted as being something that wouldn't take off when invented in 1816. We should not dismiss what may be deemed as 'low tech', as it may actually remain more significant in aiding older people in their self-care. Tools such as the grabber stick, full page magnifying window, big button and amplified telephone, the 'talking' blood glucose meter and the jar opening tools and more should not be forgotten. Just because something is new, doesn't mean it is better.

9.11   Chapter Summary

Person-centred diabetes care today necessitates HPs to be innovative and to personalise care with each individual. The speed of technological change is driving healthcare towards more digital solutions. HPs should ensure they are actively aware of the ongoing developments and resources available and that we have them in the growing toolbox of support that can assist the older person with diabetes.

The only thing that is constant is change—(Heraclitus 500BC).

Key Points for Readers to Reflect on

- Reflect on how you currently support the use of technology for older people with diabetes.
- Do you talk about technology in your consultations and/or education programs?
- What technologies are you familiar with. Are they likely to benefit older people with diabetes care?
- How would you know/find out?
- Are you up-to-date in your understanding of technology in diabetes care?

9.12 Further Resources

- The new mobile age: How technology can extend the healthspan and optimize the lifespan. Joseph Kvedar MD (to be published Oct 2017)
- Christopher Kelly—Using Machine Learning for Health, The Paleo Solution Podcast—Robb Wolf. Episode 369 18th July 2017
- The wonderful and terrifying implications of computers that can learn. Jeremy Howard, TED Talk. Ted.Com Dec 16 2014.

References

Anderson M, Perring A (2017). Pew Research Center: tech adoption climbs among older adults. Pew Research Center. Available at http://www.pewinternet.org/2017/05/17/tech-adoption-climbs-among-older-adults/. Accessed 13 Oct 2017

Australian Bureau of Statistics (2016) Household Use of Information Technology, Australia, 2014–15. cat. no. 8146.0. Available at http://www.abs.gov.au/AUSSTATS/abs@.nsf/allprimarymainfeatures/ACC2D18CC958BC7BCA2568A9001393AE?opendocument. Accessed 13 Oct 2017

Bouma H, Fozard JL, Van Bronswijk JEMH (2009) Gerontechnology as a field of endeavour. Gerontechnology 8(2):68–75

Chen M, Ma Y, Song J, Lai CF, Hu B (2016) Smart clothing: Connecting human with clouds and big data for sustainable health monitoring. Mobile Netw Appl 21(5):825–845. https://doi.org/10.1007/s11036-016-0745-1

Chesters J, Ryan C, Sinning M (2013) Older Australians and the take-up of new technologies. National Centre for Vocational Education Research

Chow CK, Redfern J, Hillis GS, Thakkar J, Santo K, Hackett ML, Jan S, Graves N, de Keizer L, Barry T, Bompoint S (2015) Effect of lifestyle-focused text messaging on risk factor modification in patients with coronary heart disease: a randomized clinical trial. JAMA 314(12):1255–1263. https://doi.org/10.1001/jama.2015.10945

Diabetes Prevention Program (DPP) Research Group (2002) The diabetes prevention program (DPP). Diabetes Care 25(12):2165–2171. https://doi.org/10.2337/diacare.25.12.2165

Feist H, McDougall K (2013) Older people's use of new communication technologies: research findings and policy implications. Aust Popul Migration Res Centre Policy Brief 1(8):1–7

Furlong M (1995) Communities for seniors in cyberspace. Ageing Int 22(1):31–33

Holmes J (2011). Why texting is the most important information service in the world. New America Foundation. Available at http://www.theatlantic.com/technology/archive/2011/08/why-texting-is-the-most-important-information-service-in-the-world/242951/. Accessed 12 Oct 2017

How to Further Integrate Patient-Facing Apps in Healthcare (and the Top-Rated Apps)' (2013). Available at: https://www.beckershospitalreview.com/healthcare-information-technology/how-to-further-integrate-patient-facing-apps-in-healthcare-and-the-top-rated-apps.html. Accessed 13 Oct 2017

Jakicic JM, Davis KK, Rogers RJ, King WC, Marcus MD, Helsel D, Rickman AD, Wahed AS, Belle SH (2016) Effect of wearable technology combined with a lifestyle intervention on long-term weight loss: the IDEA randomized clinical trial. JAMA 316(11):1161–1171

Kassavou A, Sutton S (2017) Automated telecommunication interventions to promote adherence to cardio-metabolic medications: meta-analysis of effectiveness and meta-regression of behaviour change techniques. Health Psychol Rev:1–18. https://doi.org/10.1080/17437199.2017.1365617

Kemp S (2017). Digital in 2017 global overview (2017). *We Are Social & Hootsuite*.

Lally P, van Jaarsveld CHM, Potts HWW, Wardle J (2010) How are habits formed: modelling habit formation in the real world. Eur J Soc Psychol 40:998–1009

Leavengood LB (2001) Older people and Internet use. Generations 25(3):69–71

Magnusson L, Hanson E, Borg M (2004) A literature review study of information and communication technology as a support for frail older people living at home and their family carers. Technol Disabil 16(4):223–235

McCurry J (2015) Japan will be model for future super-ageing societies. Lancet 386(10003):1523

Neubeck L, Lowres N, Benjamin EJ, Freedman SB, Coorey G, Redfern J (2015) The mobile revolution [mdash] using smartphone apps to prevent cardiovascular disease. Nat Rev Cardiol 12(6):350–360

Nouchi R, Taki Y, Takeuchi H, Hashizume H, Akitsuki Y, Shigemune Y, Sekiguchi A, Kotozaki Y, Tsukiura T, Yomogida Y, Kawashima R (2012) Brain training game improves executive functions and processing speed in the elderly: a randomized controlled trial. PLoS One 7(1):e29676. https://doi.org/10.1371/journal.pone.0029676

Pew Research Center (2012) Older adults and internet use. Available at: http://pewinternet.org/Reports/2012/Older-adults-and-internet-use.aspx. Accessed 13 Oct 2017

Piwek L, Ellis DA, Andrews S, Joinson A (2016) The rise of consumer health wearables: promises and barriers. PLoS Med 13(2):e1001953. https://doi.org/10.1371/journal.pmed.1001953

Quinn CC, Shardell MD, Terrin ML, Barr EA, Ballew SH, Gruber-Baldini AL (2011) Cluster-randomized trial of a mobile phone personalized behavioural intervention for blood glucose control. Diabet Care 34(9):1934–1942

Ramachandran A, Snehalatha C, Ram J, Selvam S, Simon M, Nanditha A, Shetty AS, Godsland IF, Chaturvedi N, Majeed A, Oliver N (2013) Effectiveness of mobile phone messaging in prevention of type 2 diabetes by lifestyle modification in men in India: a prospective, parallel-group, randomised controlled trial. Lancet Diabet Endocrinol 1(3):191–198

Simons DJ, Boot WR, Charness N, Gathercole SE, Chabris CF, Hambrick DZ, Stine-Morrow EA (2016) Do "brain-training" programs work? Psychol Sci Public Interest 17(3):103–186. https://doi.org/10.1177/1529100616661983

Singh K, Drouin K, Newmark LP, Rozenblum R, Lee J, Landman A, Pabo E, Klinger EV, Bates DW (2016) Developing a framework for evaluating the patient engagement, quality, and safety of mobile health applications. Issue Brief (Commonw Fund) 5(1):11

Smith A (2014) Older adults and technology use: adoption is increasing, but many seniors remain isolated from digital life. Pew Research Center. Available at http://www.pewinternet.org/files/2014/04/PIP_Seniors-and-Tech-Use_040314.pdf. Accessed 13 Oct 2017

Stokke R (2016) The personal emergency response system as a technology innovation in primary health care services: an integrative review. J Med Internet Res 18(7)

Tegart G (2010). Smart Technology for Health Longevity. Report of a study by the Australian Academy of Technological Sciences and Engineering (ATSE)

The Conversation (2017). Robot revolution: why technology for older people must be designed with care and respect, Feb 1, 2017.Available at http://theconversation.com/robot-revolution-why-technology-for-older-people-must-be-designed-with-care-and-respect-71082. Accessed 13 Oct 2017

Victorian Health Promotion Foundation (2013). Technology and older people: findings from the VicHealth Indicators Survey. 15th Oct, 2013. Available at: http://apo.org.au/node/36000. Accessed 13 Oct 2017

World Health Organization (2015) World report on ageing and health. World Health Organization

Personalised Care and Research

10

David Strain

> *I would never allow a scientist to partake in government;*
> *Give them a new piece of information and they are liable to*
> *change their mind*
>
> *(Abraham Lincoln 1809–1865)*

Key Points

- Diabetes management is a rapidly changing environment
- Older adults are routinely excluded from clinical trial programs
- Evaluation of the results of clinical trials and the applicability to the population that we work with is a skill in its own right
- This chapter details a systematic approach to evaluating data from these clinical trials and how to apply it to the population that we work with.
- Finally, it will review the difference between personalisation and individualisation in the application of treatments to improve outcomes for the people with diabetes

10.1 Introduction

When Abraham Lincoln made the statement on the previous page he was in a rapidly changing political environment, leading his country through a Civil War, the abolition of slavery, an evolution of the federal government and modernisation of the economy. He required stability from his government in a changing landscape, and quipped that the scientist could not provide stability on a background of ever-changing evidence. It is rather ironic, therefore, that today we live in a changing medical environment, with the number of people with diabetes approximately quadrupling over the last 30 years and advances in the evidence base occurring on an almost daily basis, yet we healthcare scientists find ourselves in a state of inertia continuing to do what we have always done, because "that's the way we do things".

D. Strain
University of Exeter Medical School, Exeter, UK
e-mail: D.Strain@exeter.ac.uk

© Springer International Publishing AG, part of Springer Nature 2018
T. Dunning (ed.), *The Art and Science of Personalising Care with Older People with Diabetes*, https://doi.org/10.1007/978-3-319-74360-8_10

By reading this book, you have committed to the first step to change your own practice working with older adults who have diabetes, however, now your biggest challenge begins—how do you apply the evidence cited in the book and guidelines and other clinical recommendations? An even greater future trial will follow. Almost by definition, even if first publication of new research coincides with publication of the book, the book will be out-of-date the day you purchased it.

10.2 How Do We Integrate Tomorrow's Evidence with Today's Learnings?

Paradoxically, applying evidence to the people we work with is increasingly becoming less of a science and more of an art. The first step towards applying evidence-based medicine is evaluating the relevance of new information to our population. Older adults are routinely excluded from trials in diabetes. In one review, 65% of clinical trials in diabetes had an arbitrary upper age limit (Cruz-Jentoft et al. 2013) for no specified reason. Of the remaining studies, 77% of trials exclude people on basis of "co-morbidities", 30% of trials exclude them on the basis of polypharmacy, 18% exclude those with cognitive impairment and 9% exclude those with a short life expectancy. Indeed, only 1.4% of studies specifically included older adults. Therefore, due to the sparsity of evidence in the older adults we are often left to review, evaluate, extrapolate and implement from studies in younger populations. This is only an issue if there are significant age-based differences in the response to the intervention in populations based on how long they walked the earth. Unfortunately, there are, indeed, significant differences between the responses to therapies between the more mature and the young.

The differences in physiology between a healthy adult at the age of 65 and an older adult, at the age of 80 years, are greater than those occurring between a toddler and a teenager progressing to adulthood. For the latter, with the exception of the secondary sexual characteristics, the difference is purely size and the ability to throw a good tantrum, whereas for the ageing adult there are fundamental changes in the way the heart, kidneys, brain, liver, endothelium, autonomic nervous system, indeed, just about every system in the body, respond to external stimuli in the later years of life (see Chap. 1). Simple examples include the optimal blood pressure, which rather than the 130/80 target that we aim for with younger adults sits at approximately 150/90 (Delgado et al. 2017).

Indeed, in the real world, an 85-year-old adult on antihypertensive therapy at the conventional target 130/80 has a similar mortality to a person with a blood pressure at 180/110. Whereas, the latter value would undoubtedly trigger a therapeutic intervention, it would not be conventional practice to deprescribe anti-hypertensives for the former. Similarly, our conviction that obesity is an adverse prognostic indicator is equally misconceived in older adults, who after the age of 80, have a longer life expectancy the larger the BMI (Kamel and Iqbal 2001).

These examples may seem like a reason to maintain the status quo pending further research; indeed, there will always be an argument for more age-specific data or better and more representative trials. However, waiting for these data is often an implicit decision not to act, or to act based on past practice rather than attempting to modify our approach based on the best available evidence (Friedman et al. 2015). The goal, therefore, should be to evaluate the existing evidence in a systematic manner to determine its applicability to the population we engage with, the relevance and the potential impact of any intervention on our population. Once we have appraised all these data, we can then derive appropriate recommendations for an individual that we are working with towards improved health.

10.3   So What Do We Need to Look for in a Good Clinical Trial Report?

The first consideration should be the population studied (sampling population). Just about every scientific paper today comes with the same "Table 1, baseline characteristics". It is by far the most boring table you could look at, however at the same time it gives the most important information about the study if one asks: does the population resemble my patients? As already mentioned, however, very few studies include older adults and fewer still include frail elderly people or those with cognitive impairment; therefore in most cases this Table 1 of the manuscript that you are reviewing will alert health professionals (HP) to how much extrapolation is required.

The next question would be to consider the intervention itself. Is it tolerable or practical for older people? One must question the practicality of complex diet and exercise regimens, daily injections such as the GLP-1 receptor agonists, medications that exacerbate polyuria such as the SGLT-2 inhibitors, reduce immune responses such as the anti-inflammatory monoclonal anti-bodies, or have their impact by attenuating physiological responses such as several antihypertensive agents. In addition, consider the side-effect profile, with particular reference to their potential impact in older people with frailty or sarcopaenia. Typical examples are the risk of osteoporosis with PPARγ antagonists (thiazolidinediones; glitazones), lactic acidosis and tolerability with Metformin, the risk of candidiasis with SGLT2-inhibitors or the risk of hypoglycaemia with sulphonylureas and insulin.

Of course, having effectively dismissed every class of glucose lowering medicines as potentially harmful for many older people, the comparator medicine also requires consideration. Very often the comparator is "usual care" with the intention to maintain glycaemic equipoise. This, of course, works on the basic assumption that our current treatment strategy has a good evidence base itself. In practice, this is not necessarily the case, especially for older people. Many "traditional" therapies, such as metformin or sulphonylureas, have been in use for over 60 years, place prior to the requirement to test efficacy, or even safety. The multi-disciplinary approach to diabetes management has an evidence base of only 160 patients (Gaede et al. 2008), the only large-scale trial to test diet and exercise in people with diabetes was discontinued prematurely because of futility (LOOK AHEAD research group 2013) and, to date, only one study has even attempted to individualise care for older adults (Strain et al. 2013). Interval subsequently reported that, when asked to and given training about how to personalise glycaemic goals for frail older adults, on average, HPs set target HbA_1c of 7.0%, ignoring frailty measures, co-morbidities and poly-pharmacy in favour of considering baseline HbA_1c and local guidelines when target setting (Strain et al. 2017).

The point of asking HPs to consider these factors when evaluating comparators is not to undermine the concept of "usual care", but to stress that "usual care" is itself a heterogeneous concept, very often based on local opinion rather than rigor-ously tested protocols. This is important, because any benefit demonstrated over a strategy that you already rejected as being ineffective, does not help your quest to improve the outcomes of your partnership with the older person with diabetes.

Only now that we have considered the population, the tolerability and appropri-ateness of the intervention and the suitability of the comparator should we turn to look at the results. But, divergent to most evidence evaluation protocols, our next point of call is the subgroup analyses, usually figure or Table 2. This is in contrast to the usual practice of considering the magnitude of benefit of the intervention itself; however, without an approximation of the applicability of the results to our population the context of any benefit cannot be estimated.

Subgroup analyses should only ever be regarded as hypothesis generating, but, in the absence of good age-specific data, our entire practice is based on hypothesising which interventions will provide the most benefit, whilst with the least risk of side effects. The specific subgroup analysis of interest will be exploring the results in the different age groups within the study. Typically, there will be an analysis with an arbitrary cut-off around the age of 65. If this suggests that the benefit is at least mir-rored in the older subgroup, it is reasonable to assume that any benefit may be extrapolated into older populations than studied. Conversely, if the benefit is attenu-ated in the older population within the study, we should be cautious of generalising the results to the more mature population that we see daily.

10.4 Aligning These Results with the Person in Front of Us

If the data meet these tests, our next step is to explore the magnitude and time scale of benefit, notably whether we could anticipate a benefit to our patient beyond their current therapy during their anticipated life expectancy. An intervention which starts to show benefit at 9 years and achieves significance at 16 has very little rele-vance to a 92-year-old patient (unless they are indeed worried about their risk of stroke at the age of 108!)

Determining potential benefit is a skill all on its own. Clinical trials often present relative risk reduction, absolute risk reduction, numbers needed to treat, odds ratios or hazard ratios. I could write a book considering the relative merit of these alone, however suffice it to say that for our purposes, there are two values that we are par-ticularly interested in. The first is the risk of an event in the control population, often hidden in the results table as the percentage of outcomes in the placebo or usual care group. This gives us a denominator that we can scale up or down according to the risk of outcomes in our population. If at all possible, we should only consider non-fatal outcomes. Although a controversial step, one inescapable fact is that we will never prevent a death, despite what some studies, particularly those sponsored by pharmaceutical companies, may have us believe.

Every person we treat will die…. eventually. We are in the business of working with older adults to improve the quality of their remaining years rather than increasing the quantity, thus outcomes associated with improved quality of life, such as non-fatal stroke, hospitalisations or visual loss, are more pertinent. The second figure we need to know is the relative risk reduction (RRR). From this we can calculate an absolute risk reduction and number needed to treat to inform our conversations when choosing treatments.

If, for example, a study reports the risk of stroke in their control population was 8%, and intervention X reduced this by 25% (RRR), this tells us that in the study it actually reduced the risk of stroke by 2% (i.e. 25% of 8%). This means that for every 50 people given the treatment, we would prevent 1 stroke (referred to as the number needed to treat (NNT); calculated as 100/absolute risk reduction = 100/2 = 50). However, we know in our older population the actual risk of a stroke is closer to 24%, due to their advancing age and multiple co-morbidities. Therefore, a RRR reduction of 25% would translate to a 6% absolute risk reduction (25% of 24%) and us only having to treat 17 people to prevent a stroke (NNT; 100/6).

Clearly this isn't great for the 16 who took the tablet but weren't going to get a stroke anyway, but in the absence of a reliable prognostic indicator (or crystal ball), this is inevitable, and with odds like this combined with only 1 in 100 getting any side effects of note, a very easy conversation to have. Another intervention with a very similar side-effect profile may reduce the risk of sight threatening retinopathy by the same 25% from the same 8% baseline risk. In this case, however, we know that age-related macular degeneration is of much greater risk that true diabetic retinopathy, and actually diabetes only accounts for approximately 2% of vision loss in elderly people. That translates to a 0.5% absolute risk reduction, 200 patients exposed to prevent one experiencing a significant deterioration in sight. We are now left saying for every person whose eyes we protect we cause two people significant harm, and the remaining 197 have just endured the minor inconvenience of two more tablets a day, slight GI disturbance, but absolutely no benefit. A completely different conversation is required during our consultation.

These calculations of number needed to treat and numbers needed to harm lead to the most difficult component of applying personalised medicine, where the real art is required. Once we have evaluated the evidence, accepted its validity, extrapolated the potential benefits and decided that we believe that the new intervention has the potential to benefit the person in front of us, we now have to evaluate the person we are with to determine what is the right therapy for them.

10.5 Who Are We Working with—A Participant, an Individual or a Person?

A clinical trial works in a perfect, somewhat sterile environment. The population are selected primarily based on their suitability to participate in the trial, notably their ability to adhere to treatment regimens. Indeed, medication adherence in clinical trials is usually in the region of 95%, whereas in clinical practice only approximately a third of our patients take at least 80% of their medication. Before you mentally castigate all those people with diabetes for not looking after themselves, or dismiss the figures because "all of my patients take all of their tablets" ask yourself have you, or anyone close to you, ever been prescribed a single course of antibiotics for any reason, but stopped taking them after about 3 days when you started to feel better, despite the doctor's advice to complete the course…

Additionally, the results of any clinical trial represent effects at a population level, not the benefit to an individual. One cannot prevent a third of a stroke or two-fifths of a heart attack, therefore we must individualise the choices and advise accordingly, working with the person. Throughout this book we have been talking about the varying special considerations for our older adults; cognitive decline, multi-morbidity, renal impairment, polypharmacy, each regarded as a separate entity. The reality, however, is that each rarely occurs in isolation. Therefore, when assessing the applicability of the research to the person we are working with towards better health, we must not only consider the potential risks and benefits of the prospective intervention, but also the potential natural history for the individual. Prognostication is never an exact science, however, in order to best advise our patients, we must try to anticipate the complications most likely to afflict them. We can then advise as to the best opportunities to maintain their health. This relationship is integral to our ability to improve their outcomes. Indeed, only when the HP, the people with diabetes and their carers or family work together as a team can the health outcomes for the individual be optimised (Strain et al. 2014). Communication is the key to improving adherence to therapy, indeed, in my mind at least. Communication makes the difference between individualised care and personalised care.

- *Individualisation* is the process of considering all of the variables that make a person we are caring for a complex multi-morbid case, establishing appropriate therapeutic targets and developing a treatment strategy to achieve these targets.
- *Personalisation* is the process of considering the factors of importance to the person we are working with in order to achieve a maintenance of specific health goals.

Although these are aligned, they are not the same. For example, the individualised target may be to maintain glycaemic control at a value that will reduce the risk of progressive retinopathy, whereas the personalised target would be to facilitate our patient clearly seeing their grandchild graduate in 4 years time. In order to realise the personalised goal, we would need to achieve the individualised targets. However, a mutual understanding of the person's goal will help the HP understand the individualised targets. We hope personalised care will lead to improved medication adherence and thus improve the person's chances of achieving both goals. Chapter 2 discusses personalised care and shared decision-making and Chap. 3 discusses the characteristics HPs need to be able to personalise care with older people.

10.6 National Health Service—Adding More Life to the Years or

10.6.1 National Disease Service—Fighting the Blaze Without a Fire Door in Sight

Of course, here is the biggest problem with preventative medicine. Nobody will ever truly see the benefit of good glycaemic and blood pressure control or good adherence with statin therapy, for the real benefit will be in the strokes, myocardial infarctions and amputations that *do not* occur. No patient would ever know the potential impact of not taking their therapy, they only see what actually happens. Therefore, if their vision does marginally deteriorate or they suffer a transient ischaemic attack (TIA), it may be difficult to convince them that this is not treatment failure, but actually a measure of the success of the good decisions that they have made. Without these interventions, the marginal deterioration in vision may have been total blindness; the TIA, a large ischaemic stroke with devastating consequences.

10.6.2 Collaborative Healthcare with the Person at the Centre

Personalised goal setting, therefore, is a route to improving collaboration between patient and healthcare practitioner. Appropriate communication between the healthcare practitioner, the person with diabetes and their personal support network, whether that be family or carers, allows elucidation of that which is most important to them. For many this may not be related to diabetes at all, for others it may be a fear of visual loss, stroke whilst others still may be more worried about the risks of hypoglycaemia. The knowledge of this may help you work with a patient towards achieving this goal. Unfortunately, only approximately 50% of the people we see appreciate that the purpose of the therapy is to reduce the risk of complications at all (Strain et al. 2014).

The remainder believe that the aim is to chase glycaemic targets, hit numerical values or simply take the tablets because the "doctor told me to…" With this level of basic knowledge, it is not surprising that tablet adherence is low, dietary adjustments are short-lived and lifestyle changes are not even attempted. For only when the person with diabetes understands the purpose of their treatment can they comply with the complex regimens that we suggest to them. Only by personalising the explanations of the treatment options, can we achieve the individualised goal. How many of us write on the box "to control blood pressure", "to reduce cholesterol", or "to regulate high blood sugars"? Surely "Prevent a stroke", "Stop a heart attack" and "avert blindness" would have greater impact.

10.6.3 Can It Work vs. Does It Work; the RCT vs. the Real World

There is one final, major consideration before handing out any prescription. So far throughout this book, each chapter has considered existing interventions in isolation towards various individual goals. This final chapter has dealt with how to integrate new therapeutics into our armamentarium. However, there remains a significant hole in our knowledge as to the implementation of personalised care in older adults. This data deficit, however, is fuelled by the perception that research is performed by career academics sat in their ivory towers devising cunning trial strategies. If these academics were truly interested in the person with diabetes they would be on the front line "doing" rather than in the general's quarters "planning". Historically this may have been the case, but today's research has a different appearance. There have been a multitude of studies gauging *can* an intervention work. This is the hallmark of the pharmaceutical sponsored, placebo controlled, prospective randomised interventional trial. In addition to the active drug or a placebo, each participant gets a support plan, additional dietetics and lifestyle advice, far more frequent monitoring and access to a motivated research team to ensure that good adherence is met for the duration of the study. In today's healthcare system, given the global financial situation, there is a growing demand on research to establish *does* it work. This requires a different far more pragmatic approach to research. And this is often best done by people like you.

10.6.4 Answering Tomorrows' Questions

You will have opportunities to shape the research that takes place in your centre whether through choosing appropriate studies to participate in or developing your own protocols. There is a significant hole in the data regarding the care of older adults, notably whether personalisation of care is even worth it. After all, personalised care takes additional time. Time is a very precious resource within any healthcare system. If one was to introduce any intervention, we would expect a risk/benefit and cost-effectiveness analysis to be performed to ensure good value is being achieved. It is, therefore, only reasonable that if you want to implement any change in practice, whether that be a drug, a new diet, a lifestyle intervention, or simply spending an extra 20 min with the person with diabetes establishing their wants and needs and agreeing strategies to achieve these goals that we justify our actions by auditing our outcomes. This is the very heart of the most relevant research to our practice. *Does what we do matter?*

At the time of writing, there has only been one published study exploring individualised targets in older adults, and that only had limited success. The *Individualised Treatment targets for Elderly people with type 2 diabetes using Vildagliptin Add-on or Lone therapy (INTERVAL)* study aimed to set individualised goals for people over the age of 70 with type 2 diabetes. Unlike many studies even in older adults there were no restrictions for participation, other than the ability to give informed consent. As a result, there were frail, in some cases institutionalised, participants. Investigators were asked to discuss individualised targets with each potential participant; consider frailty, co-morbidities, polypharmacy, baseline characteristics and local guidance, then establish individualised glycaemic targets for each person. There were two significant findings from this study. The first is the disappointing observation that, even with appropriate training and freedom beyond any local incentives or penalties, local experts in treating diabetes in older adults still set an average HbA_1c target of 7.0% (53 mmol/mol) in keeping with local guidelines. This may have been due to the confidence of the practitioners in the agent that was being used and its low risk of hypoglycaemia; however it was more likely that practitioners still do not feel confident to step outside of their comfort zone. There is a significant inertia in medicine, not just in the escalation of therapy but also in moving away from conventional targets and guidelines set based on historic research findings.

The other, far more promising result, was that the consultation alone enabled 27% of participants treated only with placebo achieved their individualised goal. This is despite providing no additional support, dietary or lifestyle advice, and specifically asking participants not to further adjust their behaviours, other than to take the medication or it's matched placebo. By virtue of their registering for and participating in a clinical trial, these were likely to be the already more motivated individuals, and yet with only one conversation where physicians attempted to personalise their diabetes care, over a quarter hit individualised targets. Our favoured explanation for this is that given the chance to discuss their diabetes and consider their priorities individuals felt more empowered to manage their own disease.

There are of course many other potential theories to explain this benefit, improved adherence to medication, prompting towards targets, the act of observation changing the behaviours of that which is observed, known in research as the Hawthorne effect (actually named after the Hawthorne Electrical Works in Cicero Illinois. During a study of different levels of factory lighting, it was noted that having researchers actively monitoring working and break patterns increased productivity amongst employees, irrespective of the change to the lights. Mayo and Landsberger independently concluded that the act of holistically considering the worker as a person and the novelty of being a research subject improved output. Neither considered that having the boss watch what you're doing, right at the start of the Great Depression of 1929–30, would increase motivation engendered by a lack of job security, but that's researchers for you.

However, each of these (the adherence, prompting and observation, not the lights or depression) is predicated on the fact that older adults actively participate in clinical trials. When asking investigators how they perceive research with older adults, there will be many preconceptions on the limitations of their ability to participate in clinical trials. Many of these are false, indeed, in my experience working with older adults is not only more rewarding but actually easier than working with the relative youngsters under the age of 65.

Just exploring some of these so-called limitations in detail.

1. *It's difficult to get them to participate.*

Erm… to be polite, nonsense! In the INTERVAL study, the projected 18-month recruitment period, based on extrapolations from studies in younger cohorts, was halved to 9 months when all targets were met ahead of schedule. Older adults *want* to participate, whether that be to gain an increase sense of worth, to "give something back", or simply because they want to partake in active research. In every study that I have been involved with, whether as chief investigator, local principle investigator or simply as the "hands on the ground", I have found it easier to recruit and retain older adults than those under the age of 65, indeed in a recent 2400 participant cohort, not only did we recruit ahead of schedule, but those who were unable to partake were actively seeking alternative studies when they were told recruitment was complete.

2. *They are already too sick.*

Surely that is the point. Older adults are more likely to have co-morbidities and be exposed to polypharmacy. This is, however representative of the majority of people around the world with type 2 diabetes. In a rigorously conducted, randomised controlled trial, these co-morbidities are balanced between arms. Further, in the multi-morbid populations, outcomes and adverse events are more likely to occur. When a clinical trial is powered on a reduction in number of events between populations, a higher frequency of complications from the diabetes increases the power of the study to detect differences between the intervention and usual care.

3. *They are incapable of following instructions and taking tablets*

This is very difficult to quantify, but the evidence would suggest the absolute converse is true. Age is the single strongest predictor of medication adherence in the general population such that the older the patient, the more likely they are to take their medications as directed. Age-specific adherence figures in clinical trials have never been reported, however there is no reason to believe that those motivated enough to join in a clinical trial should for some reason be less motivated to participate than the general population, indeed my experience suggests that the absolute converse is true, and it is incredibly unusual to have an elderly trial participant with less than 95% medication adherence.

4. *They're all in nursing homes and can't come to the study clinic*

A popular misconception; that is often held not only by those planning clinical trials, but also purchasers and service providers. Unfortunately, this myth is perpetuated by the media, who choose to represent the elderly as infirm, often with significant care needs, in keeping with the old "mother-in-law" jokes. The reality, however, is less than 5% of the elderly population are in any sort of institutional care. The majority are completely independent and living a very active life.

From a clinical trial standpoint, their retirement often makes them more willing subjects, affording them more flexibility when planning their study visits around their social activities rather than a work schedule. Occasionally this can be a paradoxical problem—as I type I am trying to schedule a 78-year-old gentleman's study visits around his weekly golf tournaments, twice weekly bowling club, tennis and poker evenings. Whereas the poker evenings themselves do not cause scheduling conflicts, the requirement to be abstinent from alcohol renders the following day unsuitable.

The reality is research with older adults is an absolute pleasure. They are undoubtedly the most motivated cohort to work with and also considerably more representative of the general population with diabetes. I write this not only to show pride in what we do, but also to inspire. As you come to the end of the chapter and the book, and congratulations for making it this far, we have discussed a multitude of different strategies for personalising care for the older adults that we work with. You have read the opinions and interpretation of the evidence of a collection of experts in their fields. You may disagree with some of the opinions expressed, most likely in the areas that you too are an expert in.

The fact remains, however, that there are very few "facts" in the personalisation of care. Facts such as if you give drug X you will achieve a HbA_1c reduction of 0.7% or 8 mmol/mol are nice, but they are of little relevance when the actual personalisation takes place determining whether it is worthwhile to reduce average glycaemia by this amount in the first place. At the moment, there is no fixed way to personalise care. Everyone does it slightly differently, and everyone believes their way is slightly better—otherwise they would have adapted and taken on the patterns of someone else. The biggest research area in the future of diabetes management will be not some new molecule that can bind to a new receptor on the surface of a particular cell type, but the development and validation of pathways that can ensure each patient gets the right treatment to help them achieve their own goal.

And the best people to do this research:—you and the people with diabetes that you work with. Standardise your approach, monitor the successes, and the failings, then report what worked so that others can build on your successes.

10.7 Chapter Summary

Older adults are often not included in clinical research programmes, and, because of the fundamental differences in the physiology of older adults, careful consideration must be made before extrapolating existing and emerging evidence onto an elderly cohort. We have discussed a systematic process to evaluate new information using a modified PICO (Patient, Intervention, Control and Outcome relevance) approach. We can use this method to determine the applicability of the research and the outcomes demonstrated to the population that we treat. Further, we have considered the merits of alternative sources of evidence from the traditional randomised controlled trial, specifically pragmatic study design and real-world data. Although often decried by academics, these strategies can often provide more useful information when attempting to personalise care. The contrast between personalised care, which establishes what is important to the person with diabetes and individualised goal setting, which focuses on the numerical targets that may need to be attained in order to achieve the personalised ambitions. We have discussed the perceived barriers to including older adults in clinical trials, dismissing each obstacle in turn. Finally, we have established that there is a dearth of good evidence for how best to personalise care, and that any reports, no matter how small can only improve the overall landscape, therefore we would urge you as an active practitioner to consider standardising your approach and publish your results.

10.8 Reflection Points

- The fundamental physiological differences in older adults should not be underestimated when considering the suitability of a new intervention.
- Practice the modified PICO evaluation on all manuscripts that may alter your approach to managing an older person with diabetes.
- Personalised care and individualised goal setting are not the same:
  - Personalised care identifies what is important to a person and how we can best meet that person's ambitions.
  - Individualised care establishes the targets or goals that we may need to reach to achieve those ambitions.
- You can shape the future research of optimising diabetes care in older adults by developing and participating in trial programs, enrolling patients, or just establishing what you do well and talking about it.

References

Cruz-Jentoft AJ, Carpena-Ruiz M, Montero-Errasquín B, Sánchez-Castellano C, Sánchez-García E (2013) Exclusion of older adults from ongoing clinical trials about type 2 diabetes mellitus. J Am Geriatr Soc 61(5):734–738

Delgado J, Masoli JAH, Bowman K, Strain WD, Kuchel GA, Walters K, Lafortune L, Brayne C, Melzer D, Ble A, As part of the Ageing Well Programme of the NIHR School for Public Health Research, England (2017) Outcomes of treated hypertension at age 80 and older: cohort analysis of 79,376 individuals. J Am Geriatr Soc 65(5):995–1003

Friedman SM, Shah K, Hall WJ (2015) Failing to focus on healthy aging: a frailty of our discipline? J Am Geriatr Soc 63(7):1459–1462

Gaede P, Lund-Andersen H, Parving HH, Pedersen O (2008) Effect of a multifactorial intervention on mortality in type 2 diabetes. N Engl J Med 358(6):580–591

Kamel HK, Iqbal MA (2001) Body mass index and mortality among hospitalized elderly patients. Arch Intern Med 161(11):1459–1460

Strain WD, Lukashevich V, Kothny W, Hoellinger MJ, Paldánius PM (2013) Individualised treatment targets for elderly patients with type 2 diabetes using vildagliptin add-on or lone therapy (INTERVAL): a 24 week, randomised, double-blind, placebo-controlled study. Lancet 382(9890):409–416

Strain WD, Cos X, Hirst M, Vencio S, Mohan V, Vokó Z, Yabe D, Blüher M, Paldánius PM (2014) Time to do more: addressing clinical inertia in the management of type 2 diabetes mellitus. Diabetes Res Clin Pract 105(3):302–312

Strain WD, Agarwal AS, Paldánius PM (2017) Individualizing treatment targets for elderly patients with type 2 diabetes: factors influencing clinical decision making in the 24-week, randomized INTERVAL study. Aging (Albany NY) 9(3):769–777

You have not done enough, you have never done enough, so long as it is still possible for you to have something of value to contribute

(Dag Hammmeskjold)

T. Dunning (ed.), *The Art and Science of Personalising Care with Older People with Diabetes*, https://doi.org/10.1007/978-3-319-74360-8